The Natural Organic Beauty Book

The
Natural Organic
Beauty Book

BY

GARY NULL and Staff

THE HEALTH LIBRARY

Robert Speller & Sons, Publishers, Inc.
New York, New York 10010

CONTENTS

The Natural Organic Beauty Book

INTRODUCTION

A glance at the dictionary should convince any woman that "beauty" and "glamour" are quite different things, yet men are attracted by them both.

"Beauty" is defined as "the quality of being very pleasing as in color, form and tone" while "glamour" is described as "seeming mysterious allure; bewitching charm."

All women have it within their power to look either beautiful or glamorous (but not necessarily both). By the investment of a small fortune anyone can be made glamorous by Hollywood or Fifth Avenue or Parisian experts. Wigs, gowns, plastic surgery, make-up and subtle lighting can make the most prosaic-looking woman look "glamorous." If she is willing to pay the twin prices —first for the cosmetics, clothes and advisors, then for the destruction of her natural endowments—she can enter the world of glamour and sophistication most teenage girls dream about.

Everyone knows this, and not everyone can afford it nor thinks it is the best way to live. But what so many women do not know is that they have it within their power to look *naturally* healthy and full of vitality and to exude a natural beauty. Magic potions are not necessary. All it takes is a realization that it is possible followed by a genuine desire to follow the right path.

This information is not new; it was not just handed down from a mythical Greek Goddess in a private revelation. It is a way of beauty that your grandmothers and great-grandmothers used without a second thought! It is a way that the modern woman (of the last 70 to 100 years) has lost sight of in her quest for a quick, convenient path to the goal of physical attractiveness.

A "physically fit woman" has been described as one who:
1. Is mentally and emotionally adjusted.
2. Has a normal body size, structure and function.
3. Is free from disease.
4. Has sufficient strength to do *maximum* daily tasks without undue fatigue, and still has strength left over for emergencies.

1

So far that wouldn't seem to have much to do with "beauty." But it so happens that physical fitness is a by-product of proper eating habits and proper daily exercise. Fortunately, an additional "by-product" is natural beauty! The woman who gets sufficient exercise and eats a truly nourishing diet can't help but look vivacious. She will glow with an inner beauty that people will find irresistible.

Natural well-being involves diverse, but related elements; here are just a few:

1. skin tone
2. hair sheen
3. overall figure
4. an "alive" look in the face and eyes

How do you get all this? By eating the right foods and by getting the right amount and type of exercise. The latter is perhaps the best known to you. In the back of your mind you have always known that if you "exercise more" you'll probably be in better physical shape. But probably no one has ever sat down to tell you the specific benefits of each particular exercise for every area of your body. This book will. Furthermore it will explain conventional gymnastics as well as the Yoga approach. You may choose for yourself, although we think you will see the superiority of the latter.

What about "eating the right foods?" You may protest that you watch your calories and cholesterol and eat and drink things in particular that say "Vitamin Enriched" or "Fortified With—." But you probably have no clear idea of what use the body puts all these ingredients to, and you have been deceived by clever advertisements into thinking that you are getting nourishment when you are not.

Our food is impregnated with 2,000-3,000 chemical additives which serve no nutritional purpose. Their job is to falsify the taste or color, or to preserve the commodity from decay longer than otherwise would be possible. During the preparation of fruits and vegetables for sale they are sprayed and colored and picked before ripeness or they are artificially ripened.

Grains and milk are put through various heating processes to protect against germs while valuable vitamins and minerals are removed—to be replaced later by weaker, less nutritious artificial vitamins and minerals.

Most of what we eat today is composed of empty calories which fill you up but do nothing to help your body ward off disease and keep fit (and beautiful). Unfortunately the food not only is not nourishing, in many cases it is dangerously harmful, as you will see in the chapters on Nutrition.

What about diets? They have been the rage for a couple of generations and show no sign of slackening. One would think there must be *something* to the idea, or it would have been disproven by now. But the problem is that the "diets" don't go far enough and are based on a faulty idea of what the body needs and doesn't need.

If you were in charge of constructing a building and keeping it in good repair, and saw that you were not getting a decent day's work out of any of the 100 men on the project, would it make sense to terminate 50 of the slackers and leave the other 50 to continue piddling around (or maybe just standing around doing nothing)? Or would it make better sense to hire 25 really effective, experienced, and eager-to-work carpenters, plumbers and electricians and *then* start laying off just about all those 100 goof-offs?

Eating an improper diet (and a comparatively worthless one) for years, and then deciding to stop eating just certain foods, is like firing part of an inefficient labor force.

Actually, it would be bad enough if they just milled around the construction site doing little or no work. But the problem is that they get in the way of the few go-getters on the job and usually wind up leaning against walls and stairways that are weak, and the next thing you know, your building is falling down around you bit by bit.

Do you want trained workers at work in the house of your body or lazy house wreckers? On your decision hangs the possibilities of holding onto youth or regaining it if you have begun to lose it. Because the very same materials your body needs to hang together and resist disease and old age are the same things it needs for you to look alive and healthy!

There have been many books published on different aspects of the health and beauty problems but none until now have addressed themselves to both problems. And they are really two aspects of the same problem: eating and exercise. We don't live as close to nature as women did a hundred years ago and our diet has become devitalized and poisoned. How do we recapture the agility of the body and the glowing health that used to translate into natural beauty?

Other women have taken reducing exercises, strengthening exercises, indulged in cosmetics, and eaten health foods. You've heard about them; which way should *you* go? This book is aimed at giving you an *integrated* approach, containing the best of all four. You will learn how to care for your skin, hair and figure the *natural* way; with natural exercises, natural foods and natural cosmetic and grooming aids.

You were once a vibrant and beautiful little girl running and playing in the fresh air. Where did that beauty, verve and strength go? It's still there inside you, waiting to be called forth. So get to work!

CHAPTER ONE

AN ATTRACTIVE FIGURE,
CONTROLLED NATURE'S WAY

PHYSICAL FITNESS

One out of three grown-ups is obese or otherwise out of condition. Shocking? Of course. Until you reflect that this is a push-button age we live in. Our grandmothers had to pump water by hand for cooking, drinking and washing; she had to scrub those clothes on the washboard and wring them out by hand; she had to carry the basket to the yard and hang them on the line (bending, stooping and stretching all the while); in some places she had to chop and haul firewood for cooking as well as comfort; sweeping the living room rug required a much more vigorous movement of the arms; and ultimately someone had to beat the dust out of those rugs as they hung on a washline. Those are just a few of the ways earlier women kept in shape naturally.

Today's woman may feel she still does plenty of physical activity each day, what with driving the kids to school, shopping, cooking, making beds, etc. But she must acknowledge that things like electric washing machines and dryers, electric brooms and vacuums, gas or electric heating and city-supplied water have eliminated considerable physical exercise from her everyday life.

Doctors tell us that we have 639 muscles and 208 bones in our bodies. Each has a function in keeping that machine called "your body" working smoothly. The older we become the more we tend to sag and wilt, unless we find ways to remain active.

Since a great many of nature's methods for keeping us in shape have been eliminated from our modern lives, we have to find acceptable substitute activities or exercises. Physical Fitness has to begin with the *desire* to become healthy and to stay healthy. It will be the result of physical activity, positive health habits and the proper balance between work and play.

Before you protest that you are already engaged in a lot of activ-

5

ity around the house, reflect that it is most likely constant repetition of the same movements, using the same muscles in the same way. Many days you are tense while doing these chores. As you will see, exercise and activity are not the same thing.

WHAT EXERCISE ACTUALLY DOES

When performed regularly, proper exercise distributes your weight where it belongs and serves useful bodily purposes.

It helps you to *lose* weight which is found to be beyond the body's needs. But remember: exercise alone will not cause you to lose weight; it must be in conjunction with a good, healthy diet. Neither one works alone; it is a team effort, and you're the captain.

Regular exercise will keep your body in tip-top shape throughout your life if it is built into your daily routine.

Exercise will help you retain an attractive body, or—in time—regain one.

Exercise will improve sleep and aid your digestion, and it will help overcome nervous tension.

Lastly, but most importantly, it is the most successful means (again: in conjunction with proper diet) of preventing or retarding the degenerative diseases of later life.

How does it do all these fantastic things? By removing fatigue; by distributing nutrients to all parts of the body; strengthening the muscles and stimulating the liver; by encouraging deeper breathing and improving posture; by helping rid the body of impurities.

WHAT IT'S LIKE TO BE REALLY HEALTHY

True physical fitness means that your body is free from disease, first of all. Those hundred and one little aches and pains and problems that people take for granted in our society will all but disappear from your life.

There will be no deviation from the norms for body size, structure and functions. Your body will be as it was intended by nature to be, not as our technological society has warped it to be.

You will have the strength and endurance to perform your maximum daily tasks without undue fatigue. I stress the word "maximum." And you will have sufficient reserve strength to meet emergency demands on your body.

You will be better adjusted mentally and emotionally.

NATURE'S DANGER SIGNALS

You should be able to run or row vigorously for at least six minutes and swim for ten—covering 880 yards. Try a one mile run-and-walk. If you can do it in 15 minutes you are in good shape.

But what are some of the less obvious signals that nature sends to you to alert you that all isn't well inside your body?

- Waking up in the morning feeling tired and achy.
- Indigestion, bad breath and/or constipation.
- Frequent colds, sore throats and earaches.
- Backaches, pains in the joints (ankles, knees, hips, shoulders, neck) and aching feet.
- Difficulty in falling asleep at night.
- Development of a paunch.
- Difficulty in relaxing during the day.
- Frequent headaches.
- Twitching of the face or eyelids.
- Breathlessness from climbing ordinary stairs.
- Difficulty in remaining standing up or sitting up for more than three minutes.
- The urge for snacks between meals.
- The eating of less than three well-balanced meals in a day.
- Moodiness.
- Edginess, jitteriness, nervousness, constant worrying over insignificant things.
- The realization that most people seem to irritate you.

These situations are not intended to be normal and frequent occurrences. When they are, your body is trying to tell you something. Listen!

ARE YOU OVER- OR UNDERWEIGHT?

As a good starting point on the road to recovery, check your weight on the following charts.

Desirable Weights For Women 18-25

Height with flat heels	Small Frame	Weight in ordinary clothes Medium Frame	Large Frame
4' 10''	98-106	105-113	112-122
4 11	100-108	107-115	114-124
5 0	103-111	110-118	117-128
5 1	106-114	113-121	120-131
5 2	109-118	117-125	124-135
5 3	112-121	120-128	126-138
5 4	116-125	123-133	131-143
5 5	119-129	127-137	135-147
5 6	122-132	130-140	138-151
5 7	126-136	134-144	142-155
5 8	129-140	138-148	145-159
5 9	132-143	141-151	148-162

Based on tables prepared by Metropolitan Life Insurance Company

Desirable Weights For Women 25 and over

Height with 2-inch heels	Weight in four pounds of clothes		
4' 10''	92-98	96-107	104-119
4 11	94-101	98-101	106-122
5 0	96-104	101-113	109-125
5 1	99-107	104-116	112-128
5 2	102-110	107-119	115-131
5 3	105-113	110-122	118-134
5 4	108-116	113-126	121-138
5 5	111-119	116-130	125-142
5 6	114-123	120-135	129-146
5 7	118-127	124-139	133-150
5 8	122-131	128-143	137-154
5 9	126-135	132-147	141-158
5 10	130-140	136-151	145-163

From a table of the Public Affairs Committee, Inc.

THE IMPORTANCE OF GOOD POSTURE

Never underestimate the importance of good posture, both to your health and to your appearance. You can spend all the money you want on expensive or stylish clothes, but the effect can be ruined if they are draped over a slumped or hunched body.

Good posture announces to others how you regard yourself. When actors begin to study a role, one of the first things they try to develop is the posture and walk of the person to be portrayed. In this way they hope to project to the theater audience a hint of the person's self-esteem, which may often be at variance with that indicated by the dialogue. This contradiction is but the theatrical equivalent of the real-life situation wherein what we say about ourselves announces to the world the image we wish it to think we have of ourselves, and our posture announces what we really think of ourselves.

Observe other women's walk, for instance. Do they stride purposefully and self-confidently along, sure of who they are and where they're going? Or do they bob and mince about, slumping and shuffling? Does this one seem like a Princess moving among her subjects or more like a moving van en route to a customer? Does that one seem like a thoroughbred at the starting gate or more like a farm workhorse put out to pasture?

Research indicates that most women are weak in their arms, shoulders and upper trunk muscles, causing their shoulders to sag.

In addition, weak abdominal muscles tend to produce a protruding abdomen and tilted pelvis, inviting pain in the lower back. Alternatively, a swayback may be produced which will be aggravated by high heels, throwing the body forward.

Tall women tend to add to their posture problems by slumping in order to look shorter.

Proper posture dictates that the head be held straight with the chin level; shoulders should be down and wide, knees loose and relaxed. The stomach must be held in and kept firm, the buttocks tucked in. When standing, stand tall and keep the head, upper body and rear well-balanced and over the feet.

If you have poor posture, you will need to strengthen certain muscles and stretch others. In return, you will get the following health benefits:

- Internal organs will function properly.

- Menstrual pain will be reduced (and childbirth eased).

- Increased endurance and reduced fatigue.

- Your body will be prepared for sudden energy demands.

- Increased body-coordination and control.

- Increased speed for daily tasks.

- Increased balance and bodily flexibility.

- Increased self-confidence.

Good posture is a twenty-four hour daily task and will require determination and patience to be fully beneficial. But I think you will agree that the benefits in both health and appearance make it a worthy goal.

BEGIN BY LEARNING TO RELAX

When you feel tired, nature is sending you a faint warning signal. When you feel tension, that should be like a flashing red light, ordering you to slow down!

A quick way to relaxation of tension is, upon feeling your body tensing up, to tighten it even further. Then relax as you exhale a deep breath, slowly. That may sound as if I'm saying that the way to stop crying is to cry harder, but the analogy may not be all that far off.

Whenever an actor or actress is about to go on stage, he or she tries little relaxation tricks that they have found work best for them. The same holds true for dancers, singers and performers of any kind. There is a natural tension coming from being in that spotlight with a large audience looking at you and watching your every move and listening to your every sound. The performer *must* find a way to relieve at least part of that tension before he gets on stage, otherwise it will be communicated to the audience and will most likely interfere with his ability to perform properly. Before you start to exercise, creating controlled tension, you must relax.

Here are some suggested methods of relaxing prior to an exercise period:

• Lie down on your back, extending both arms above your head. Close your eyes and try to picture yourself on the side of a windswept hill overlooking a peaceful valley where sheep are grazing. Take a deep breath and let it out slowly.

• Take a deep breath in the same position as above, then exhale slowly, counting backward from one hundred as slowly as you can. As you master this one, the number can be reduced.

• Assume the same position as above. Imagine that your whole body is in a state of weightlessness and that you are as light as a feather. Slowly sink into a state of genuine relaxation. Repeat slowly to yourself: "G-l-i-d-e, g-l-i-d-e."

Should you find that even after the above exercises there is still an area, or several areas, of tension in your body, try one of the following exercises for specific troublespots:

Legs

Stand with one side close to a table or wall so that the hand on that side may be used for support. Swing the outside leg forward and loosely backward from the hip joint. Alternate legs several times.

Neck

Sit with the spine erect and the shoulders low. Turn your head and twist and bend your neck slowly so that you stretch first to one side and then to the other. In this way the chin touches first one collarbone and then the other. Try to look down behind you from the position of maximum stretch for a few seconds. With a little practice, the taut muscles will begin to stretch.

Never jerk or force the muscles since that will only encourage the muscle tissue to contract. Stretching must be retained for an interval of time to be effective.

Trunk

Lying on your back on the floor, hands over your head, roll over onto your face. Let the motion come from the opposite hip from the direction in which your body moves. Let your feet, head, shoulders and hands drag along behind until they are drawn over by the weight of the body. Your body should roll loosely.

Once you are in a face-down position, your body should continue to move in the same direction, this time drawn over by the lead from the far shoulder. Continue loose rolling in the same direction several times before reversing. Rest as needed.

Arms

This exercise can be done standing in an erect position, sitting on a low stool, or kneeling. Swing both arms forward and down, letting them drop during the swings so that the hands brush the thighs during each motion. Try to keep the shoulders low. Continue for several rounds without hurrying and try to maintain an easy, swinging rhythm.

Back

Lie on your back with your arms at your sides. Now raise your legs slowly, keeping them straight and curling the spine up to follow them, until the toes touch the floor beyond and behind your head. Keep your knees straight, fully stretching the hamstring muscles at the back of your thighs.

You may not be able to touch your toes to the floor at first, but a chair will do if properly placed behind your head. As you loosen up, you will bypass the chair and reach the floor. Hold this position for a few seconds.

Front

Lie on your stomach with your forehead touching the floor and your hands placed at either side of your chest. Raising your head, bend the neck backward as far as possible, completely throwing out your chin. Keep your chest close to the floor.

When your head is fully swung backward, start to contract the deep muscles of your back, slowly raising your chest. The first few times it would be advisable to support your rising thorax with your hands and gradually increase the angle between your upper arm and forearm. Later you can depend on the muscles of your back alone for raising your chest.

After you have held the position for a few seconds, start to release the spinal curve, and slowly lower your chest until the whole spine is in a horizontal line and your forehead is touching the floor as it did in the beginning of the exercise.

BASIC CONDITIONING EXERCISES

The best "calorie-burners" in order of importance are:

- Swimming.
- Running in place.
- Jumping rope.
- Vigorous walking.

As indicated earlier in this book, a person in good physical shape should be able to swim about 880 yards in about ten minutes. If you can't, that should become an objective to work toward whenever you are swimming. Unfortunately, we can't swim as often as we might like, so in lieu of that, one should try running in place 25 times, starting slow and then accelerating and tapering off. Then work up to 50, 75, 100 or 125 times.

Twisting is another basic conditioner. Place your feet wide apart and raise your arms to your sides. On the count of one, touch your left toe with your right hand, keeping knees straight and standing erect. On two, touch opposite hand and toe. Do sets of ten to begin with and gradually increase to 50 or 75 counts.

Sit-Ups are an old standby, but no less useful because of that. Lie on your back with your fingers laced behind your head. Hook your toes beneath a heavy piece of furniture (or have a partner grasp your ankles to keep them on the floor). On one, pull your body up to an erect position, thighs, calves and heels still firmly held to the floor. On two, lie down. Repeat anywhere from 5 to 20 times.

To stretch, strengthen and relax neck muscles, try the *Head Turning* exercise. Turn the head as far as easily possible to one side and count three. Look forward on the fourth count. Repeat in the other direction.

Another method of relaxing neck muscles is called *Head-Circling*. Drop the head forward and roll it to the left. Then let it roll backward, then to the right and back to the forward position. Reverse direction.

If you are trying to strengthen chest muscles or tighten the back muscles, try this: Stretch arms out to the sides at shoulder height, elbows bent, hands above the chest (palms down). Fling elbows back easily and let them spring forward. Then fling hands back, straightening your arms and let them all spring back.

For increased circulation and relief of tired back muscles, try bobbing forward from the waist with your arms hanging loosely for three counts. On the fourth count return to the starting position while turning your palms upward and reaching back with your thumbs. Pull your shoulders back and lift your chest. Do this eight times.

To trim your waistline try the *Side Bend*. Feet should be slightly apart, about the distance from one shoulder to the other, and hands on hips. On the first three counts, face forward and stretch to the left in a bobbing motion. On four, return to the starting position.

Another good one for the waist is *Trunk-Twisting*. With hands on your hips, twist your shoulders to the left, keeping the hips forward, and count to three. With each count, push harder. On the fourth count, return to the forward position. Do this four times on each side.

Coordination and balance can be improved by the *Swing and Clap* exercise. On one, swing the left leg forward and clap hands under the knee. On the second count swing the left leg backward while clapping hands in back. On four, clap hands in front. Now repeat with the right leg.

Problems with flexibility of the hip joint? Do some *Leg-Swinging*. With hands on your hips, swing left leg forward on the count of one, backward on two, forward on three, and stop on four. Alternate with the right leg.

In order to relax the upper trunk, do the *Fold & Unfold*. Drop your hands, arms, head, shoulders and trunk forward in a "folded" but relaxed position on the count of one. Unfold on the next three counts, starting at the base of the spine and attempting to feel the spine straighten segment by segment until your head is erect again. Repeat this four times.

DO's AND DONT's IN EXERCISING

DO   set aside 15-20 minutes a day for exercise and make it a habit for which you'll tolerate no exceptions. You brush your teeth every day, do your exercises too.

DON'T expect magical results overnight. It took many years for your body to deteriorate to its present condition, and it can't snap back overnight.

DO   wear shorts, leotards, slacks or other loose-fitting garments. Exercise barefoot whenever possible.

DON'T skip days; it must be *every* day.

DO   begin with warm-up exercises, then go to ones to develop strength and flexibility, and end with endurance exercises.

DON'T push yourself too far, too fast.

DO   shower after your exercise period, if possible, and have a good rubdown.

DON'T begin a vigorous exercise program until you have had a heart check-up.

DO   couple these exercises with brisk walking and other outdoor activities. And remember to breathe deeply as you move about.

REMEMBER:

Physical Fitness teachers agree that a little exercise stimulates circulation of the blood, but *too much exercise* can deplete your energy reserves. So remember to start out slowly, both as to length of time and strenuousness of the exercises, and then escalate.

And don't forget the *Slant Board*. This is an extremely relaxing, pleasant way to take the strain off the muscles and the heart and divert circulation to the head, neck and face. Start with a minute or two a day and build up to the point where you can spend twenty minutes on it. Also remember to keep it set up somewhere as a stimulant to using it. If you have to drag it out of a closet and set it up each time you want it, how long is *that* going to last?

UTILIZING ORDINARY PHYSICAL ACTIVITIES

The older you get the more necessary it will be to *create* activities which will give your muscles a workout. Improvement of your figure can best be accomplished through 15-20 minutes of exercise a day *plus* a healthy diet *and* livelier movements wherever possible in your daily activities.

- Walking to and from work or school and/or doing housework.
- Stooping to make beds.
- Sweeping floors vigorously.
- Scrubbing or handwaxing a floor or a car.
- Leaning, kneeling and squatting to dust furniture.
- Washing windows.
- Weeding flower beds.
- Reaching for and leaning into office files.

Try walking more and riding less; using stairs instead of elevators or escalators for one or two floors; pull in your stomach and buttocks and hold them firm while brushing your teeth or answering the phone. Rest, relax, and wiggle your toes and fingers at frequent intervals to relieve tension. Sit and stand tall at all times.

And remember that the exercises cannot be a now and then thing; once you've broken the habit you're lost!

WHAT ABOUT ISOMETRICS?

Isometrics are very good for what they propose to do, but they don't go far enough. They do a fine job of helping a person attain a firm, lean, and physically fit body, but they do not benefit any part of the body beyond the muscles which are exercised. There is no overall stimulation of the body through increased blood circulation, etc.

When you perform an isometric exercise, you contract a given muscle or set of muscles as hard as you can for a few seconds—no more than 5 to begin with. Each exercise is designed to benefit specific muscles. The length of time they are held may gradually be increased each week by an additional second until 12 seconds are reached.

If all you want to do is enlarge or strengthen particular muscles (your thighs or your abdomen, for instance) you might find isometrics to be a useful adjunct to other forms of exercise. It will do its work through tension faster than any other known method, including weight-lifting.

With that as an introduction, here are six examples of isometric exercises for selected areas of your body. If these benefit you and you desire more, see the additional books listed at the end of this chapter.

Bust

Stand facing the side of a door jamb. Place your cupped hands on opposite sides of the jamb, using only the fingertips for contact. Take a deep breath, lifting the chest as high as possible. Apply maximum pressure with your fingertips for five seconds and then release. Rest, and then try to repeat this exercise at arms' length from the door jamb, for a variation.

In this exercise your bust is raised because you are tightening the muscles which surround the bust. The bust itself is not made of muscle, but is supported by several.

Abdomen

Sit cross-legged on a flat surface and wrap a towel around your waist in the manner of a man's cummerbund. Reach behind you with your right hand and try to grab the left end of the towel. Do the same thing with the left hand and the right end of the towel. Take a deep breath and pull your stomach in as far as you can, as if you were trying to force it back upon your backbone. At the same time, pull the towel as tight behind your back as you can.

Waist

Stand erect and relaxed, with your feet apart. Place your hands on your hips, pressing down on the hip bone. Take a deep breath and lift your chest as high as you can for five seconds while you continue to press down on the hips as hard as you can.

This also conditions the side muscles between the waist and the shoulders, and discourages the accumulation of fat along the waist and upper sides.

Thighs

Sit on the floor with your knees straight and legs outstretched in front of you. Place a round wastebasket or a hassock (preferably 16 inches in diameter) between your ankles. Place your hands on the floor behind you, palms facing away from you, and take a deep breath. While holding the breath for five seconds, squeeze your legs together as hard as you can, trying to crush the waste basket.

In this exercise, the main pressure is on the inner thigh muscles, firming them and shaping them to eliminate thigh flab.

Neck

Place your hands on your forehead, palms inward and fingers interlocked. Take a deep breath and exert pressure by pushing forward as hard as you can with your head. This has the effect of strengthening and toning the neck muscles and also improves your posture.

Upper Arms

Stand in a doorway with your feet apart and your body relaxed. Clench your fists and raise your arms so that your fists are against the door jambs over your head. Take a deep breath and press outward with your fists, away from your body, for five seconds.

RECOMMENDED FURTHER READING:

"Beauty and Health, the Scandinavian Way," Gunilla Knutson, 1969, Avon Books.

"Have Your Baby and Your Figure, Too," Dodi Schultz, 1971, Hawthorne Books.

"A Better Figure For You," Maryhelen Vannier, 1965, Tower Publications.

Chapter Two

WHAT YOUR BODY *NEEDS* FOR NOURISHMENT

ELEMENTS OF A PROPER DAILY DIET

People who are healthy look it. People who are radiantly healthy tend to look buoyant and young. Remember that, as you struggle with yourself to find the time to exercise and—as you will learn in this chapter—come to realize the importance of exercising strict control over the fuel you feed your body.

Your automobile has a delicate, yet high-powered engine which was designed to operate on certain fuels: gasoline for the carburetor, oil for the crankcase, transmission oil for the transmission, anti-freeze for the cooling system, distilled water for the battery, and grease for all kinds of moving parts. You wouldn't dream of putting distilled water in the gas tank, now would you?

You take a chance of wrecking the cooling system if you don't put that anti-freeze in before the onset of cold weather, don't you? If you ignore the red warning light on the dashboard that tells you when your oil pressure is low or your engine is overheating most people would consider you not only a careless driver, but a foolish one.

The analogy with the human body is unfortunately not very complete for many reasons. If your car breaks down it usually won't go at all and has to go to the repair shop. The mechanics may or may not find exactly what is wrong and fix it. If they try to fool you and say they fixed it when they didn't you'll keep coming back until they (or the mechanics at another garage) fix that squeak, rattle or grinding noise or you'll get rid of the car.

Try to imagine a sleek automobile that is very powerful and versatile and which is somehow running 24 hours a day. Try to imagine that all the various fuels and lubricants must be fed into the gas tank and a small computer in that car analyzes what is coming in and sends it over various internal wires and pipes to the proper recipient: oil to the crankcase, water to the battery, anti-freeze to the radiator, etc.

19

Finally try to picture an automobile paint finish that depends on the proper functioning of that computer and that fuel in order to shine as it did when it left the factory. As long as the right fuels go into the gas tank and the car is driven adequately, the finish will never fade, the windows will never crack, the headlights will never have to be replaced, etc.

This car would be so sensitive to its internal fluids that if it is *not* getting the right ingredients, the windshield will cloud over, the roof will sag, the fenders will bulge, performance will be sluggish, you will have difficulty starting it each day, and there will be all kinds of indefinable squeaks and groans coming from its machinery.

Well, in reality your body bears a considerable resemblance to this mythical car. Your body is beautiful, powerful and versatile and at least the insides of it are working 24 hours a day. Your heart, stomach, liver, intestines, brain, bladder, etc., must operate around the clock. You do receive just about all your fuels through a single point of entry (the mouth), they do go to a "gas tank" (the stomach), and a "computer" (the brain) determines the ultimate use of each ingredient.

You may *not* be aware of the further similarities in the dependency of the finish, windshield and headlights on the quality and quantity of the fuels consumed. This chapter will go into this aspect at length. We shall also discuss what happens when useless fuels are inserted and when mechanics (doctors) patch up fenders and windshields and headlights without investigating the fuel system (your diet).

VITAMINS

Vitamins were unknown prior to the early years of this century. They had existed for untold eons of time, but their existence wasn't even suspected until the turn of this century. Their existence was finally discovered through the work of Casimir Funk and Frederick G. Hopkins.

At first it was thought that there were only two vitamins, one soluble in fat, the other in water. Over the years since, many have been isolated and identified under both conditions.

These are the ones known at present:

Vitamin A
Vitamin B1 (thiamine)
Vitamin B2 (riboflavin)
Niacin
Vitamin B12
Vitamin B6   "Vitamin B Complex"
Pantothenic Acid
Folic Acid
Para-aminobenzoic Acid
Inositol
Vitamin C (Ascorbic Acid)
Vitamin D
Vitamin E
Vitamin H
Vitamin K

Vitamins have been compared to spark plugs for the body's machinery. Together with minerals they help to ignite the use of the body's fuel. Vitamins are the constituents of all living tissues. Our health is vitally dependent on their action or lack of action in the body.

As a matter of fact the word "vital" comes from the same Latin word, "vita" meaning life, as "vitamin." It would be well to remember that word origin. They are not frills to be added to the diet or ignored; they are "vital" ingredients, the lack of which will cause serious damage and deterioration to the body.

Without vitamins the body starves, yet none of them work alone. They operate as a team, mending, building, invigorating and strengthening the tissues and organs.

What about vitamin pills? Is it sufficient to take one or more vitamins via vitamin capsules (or even a "multi-vitamin")?

The problem is that Nutrition is a very new science and a great deal remains to be discovered. Once a vitamin is found, isolated and synthesized in a laboratory, it can then be mass-produced. But there are always other "ingredients" or "factors" present along with the vitamin in its natural setting which will not be present in the artificial form because no one knows about it or knows how to re-create it artificially. There is so much that we still don't know about food ingredients.

For example, experiments have shown that fish cannot live in synthetic sea water. Scientists have re-created everything analyzable in sea water, but there is something missing that hasn't yet been discovered. Because when even a small amount of genuine sea water is added to the artificial water, the fish thrive in it!

Vitamin A

- Helps vision.

- Produces a zest for living.

- Adds sheen to hair and color to skin.

- Prevents skin blemishes.

- Helps protect against infection.

- Helps protect against colds.

- Important for growth and repair of tissues.

- Plays major role in tooth formation before birth and tooth growth during infancy.

- Is found in:

Turnip greens	Carrots
Spinach	Sweet potatoes
Kale	Apricots
Broccoli	Cantaloupe
Beet greens	Pumpkin
Mustard greens	Yellow peaches
Alfalfa	Tomatoes
Asparagus	Dandelion greens
Liver	Egg yolk
Yellow cheese	Butter
Cream	Cod liver oil

Vitamin B Complex

- Needed for energy, well-being and good looks.
- Increases mental clarity.
- Acts as a natural tranquilizer.
- Helps fight fatigue and insomnia.
- Prevents beriberi.
- Fights tooth decay.
- Checks irritability.
- Helps you "get going" in the morning.
- Assists in losing unnecessary weight.
- Prevents water-storage in pregnant women and during menopause and preceding menstrual periods.
- Relieves burning feet.
- Fights epilepsy.
- Retards hair loss.
- Fights high cholesterol.
- Prevents "Morning Sickness."
- Is found in:

Brewer's yeast	Liver
Wheat germ	Yogurt
Sprouts (Soy-mung)	Whole grains
Lean pork	Lamb
Milk	Kale
Eggs	Fish
Chicken	Green peas
Green beans	Soybeans
Soybean meal	Flour
Grits	Peanuts
Spinach	Broccoli
Asparagus	Molasses
Food yeast	Sunflower seeds

Vitamin C

- Combats the common cold.

- Overcomes food poisoning.

- Stops diarrhea.

- Combats bursitis.

- Stops bleeding ulcers.

- Controls serious respiratory diseases.

- Controls bleeding gums.

- Controls post-nasal drip.

- Helps healing of wounds.

- Keeps up the body's resistance to infection.

- Is found in:

Whole oranges*	Acerola cherries
Sprouted seeds	Grapefruit
Lemon	Kumquat
Tangerines	Limes
Citron	Shaddock
Bergamot	Strawberries
Wild rose hips	Cantaloupe
Raw green foods	Tomatoes
Potatoes (white and sweet)	

*with as much of the white membrane as possible.

Vitamin D

- Strengthens bones and teeth.

- Helps teeth grow straight.

- Helps fight arthritis and bone disease (when used along with calcium or vitamin A).

- Eases menstrual pain.
- Is found in:

> Sunshine (for Spring & Summer)
> Cod liver oil (for Fall and Winter)
> Egg yolk
> Milk
> Butter
> Oily fish
> Bone meal

Vitamin E

- Builds up the heart and blood vessels.
- Builds up the reproductive system, helping childless couples to procreate after all else failed.
- Improves male virility.
- Eases menstrual and menopausal pain.
- Increases circulation.
- Dissipates moodiness.
- Improves memory.
- Helps deaden pain from sprains.
- Helps dissolve blood clots.
- Takes pain out of burns and prevents formation of scar tissue.
- Capable of removing existing scar tissue.
- Combats anemia and muscular dystrophy.
- Is found in:

> Wheat germ
> Cold pressed vegetable oils

Vitamin K

- Helps coagulate the blood.

- Is found in:

    Gelatin

    Green leafy vegetables
    (Yogurt helps your body to manufacture
    friendly bacteria in the intestinal tract).

MINERALS

Some people think of minerals as being rocks in the ground and oil and gas deposits that are mined by commercial companies for use in the business world to create things that we handle. They *are* this, but they are much, much more. Various minerals are a necessary part of our body cells and fluids. They are essential to life itself. Yet they are, to a great degree, lost during the process of refining our common everyday foods.

We must understand that there is a unity to life; a taking of life by other life, and a giving *to* life from other life. The earth, the plants, the animals and man are composed of essentially the same ingredients. We are part and parcel of the "cycle" of life.

Everyone is familiar with the water cycle, wherein the clouds drop rain onto the earth and it sinks into the ground, eventually to be drawn off into a stream which runs into a river before it empties into an ocean or lake. This water is eventually returned to the sky through evaporation in order to fulfill and resume the cycle.

There is a similar cycle in minerals. Iron, calcium, copper, prosphorus and iodine are found in the earth in large quantities and are used in mining operations. But there are also smaller quantities present in good soil. These minerals are passed on to the grass that grows on top of it; or the wheat, or fruit trees, etc.

Cows eat the grass and microscopic traces of the minerals are passed on to them; some for their own bodies' use, and others to be added to the milk they produce. We, in turn, will drink the milk, eat the beef, eat the wheat, or eat the fruit and utilize the minerals therein for our own bodily needs. And so on, throughout the cycle.

Calcium

- Regulates the heartbeat.
- Soothes the nervous system.
- Helps build strong bones and teeth.
- Is found in:

Raw milk	Skimmed milk
Natural cheese	Butter
Turnip greens	Dried peas
Beans	Bone meal
Almonds	Soybeans
Beet greens	Broccoli
Swiss chard	Cheddar cheese
Swiss cheese	Clams
Collards	Water cress
Dandelion greens	Kale
Black strap molasses	Lettuce (outer green leaves)

Phosphorus

- Helps harden the teeth by combining with calcium.
- Builds up brain tissue.
- Maintains a balance between acid and alkaline content in the blood and urine.
- Strengthens bones.
- Helps prevent rickets.
- Is found in:

Wheat	Wheat germ
Bran	Milk
Natural cheese	Egg yolk

Iron

- Feeds oxygen to every cell.

- Prevents anemia.

- Gives life to hair.

- Prevents memory loss.

- Combines with copper to form red blood cells.

- Is found in:

Liver	Leafy green vegetables
Molasses	Dried peas
Beans	Soybeans
Prunes	Eggs
Oysters	Parsley
Lentils	Beef liver

Iodine

- Creates thyroxin, a hormone which regulates the rate at which cells change oxygen and food into heat and energy.

- Prevents goiter.

- Is found in:

Seafoods	Kelp
Oysters	Sardines
Eggs	Spinach
Oatmeal	Potatoes
Milk	(with skin)
Mutton	Cabbage
Oranges	Apples

PROTEIN

Protein is what you are made of. It must be the number one diet item for healthy, happy living. Protein literally means "to come first." Every part of your body relies on protein for proper growth and normal functioning. If you have no protein, you get no proto-plasm, and thus no life!

Skin is largely protein.

Hair and fingernails are protein in different combinations.

Bones and teeth are protein in their original basic formation.

Most delicate brain and nerve tissues and blood cells are all protein in structure.

Every organ and every muscle is made of protein.

Hormones are made of protein.

Antibodies, created to fight infection, are largely protein.

No matter how much of all other foods we eat, if we don't con-sume sufficient proteins the digestive system itself won't work properly. This can be a cause of low energy (due to incomplete digestion). If you increase your proteins you will see a new bounce in your walk and a zest for life. Life gives life to life and life takes from life in order to live.

Albumin collects urine and fluid wastes from the tissues and guides them to the kidneys, lungs and skin for elimination. A lack of protein inhibits albumin from doing its job and your body will become bloated. A lot of the "fat" people carry around is just uncollected waste matter that hasn't been picked up.

Due to the American diet of refined sugar and flour, cola drinks, starchy pastry and fried foods, most of us have been living in a state of protein semi-starvation most of our lives.

Important sources of protein are:

Whole milk	Roast lamb
Calf's liver	Raw scallops
Beef liver	Eggs
Chicken liver	American cheese
Cottage cheese	Peanut flour
Powdered skimmed milk	Soybean flour
Halibut	Brewer's yeast
Stewed kidney	Dried soy beans

Sunflower seeds   Whole flour wheat
Roasted peanuts   Buckwheat flour
Peanut butter   Yellow corn meal
Unblanched almonds   Shredded wheat
Wheat germ

AMINO ACIDS

Valine. A lack of valine is indicated by awkwardness and lack of graceful movement, jittery nerves and sleeplessness.

- Source: Milk   Peanuts

Lysine. Insufficient lysine shows up in tiredness, irritability, slow growth, anemia, reproductive problems, pneumonia and bloodshot eyes.

- Source:

  Fish   Cheese
  Meat   Eggs
  Yeast   Peas
  Soybeans   Corn
  Wheat germ

Tryptophane. Necessary for the reproductive system. Lack is related to problems in that area, dry withered skin, bloodshot eyes, lost hair, and slow growth.

- Source:

  Leafy green vegetables
  Mother's milk
  Sesame seeds

Methionine. Deficiency of methionine leads to baldness, liver degeneration, and rheumatic fever.

- Source:

  Eggs   Cheese
  Sardines   Rice
  Sunflower seeds

Cystine. Utilized in glandular secretions, and helps manufacture insulin.

- Source:

Sardines	Sunflower seeds
Eggs	Cheese

Phenylalanine. Necessary for the thyroid gland. A lack is indicated by bloodshot eyes and sometimes leads to the formation of cataracts.

- Source:

Sesame seeds	Cotton seed
Oats	Cheese
Eggs	Liver

Arginine. Important to the functioning of the sex instinct in both men and women (comprising 80% of the spermatozoa). Lack of arginine leads to impotency and sterility.

- Source:

Peanuts	Sesame seeds
Peas	Eggs
Gelatin	

Glutamic Acid. Necessary for alertness and intelligence.

- Source:

All natural grains

ENZYMES

There is yet another group of proteins called enzymes. These are not to be confused with the "Enzyme Action" promised in many wash-day detergents, although the source of the word is the same.

Body enzymes are a group of proteins which act as catalysts to hasten and direct chemical reactions in living things. They exist in every cell in your body, as well as in your food. Their job is to split all foods into small bits which can be absorbed through the intestinal walls.

Unfortunately these very busy and important enzymes are very susceptible to heat. Temperatures from 50 degrees Centigrade and up for any length of time will rapidly destroy them. That's 122 degrees Fahrenheit.

Tests conducted on older people tend to show that without sufficient raw materials (from *raw* foods) the body will tire and produce fewer enzymes each year. The result of this is wrinkling of the skin, thinning of the hair, sagging muscles and lackluster eyes.

But by supplying your body with proteins, minerals, enzymes and vitamins from raw foods you may prolong health, youth and life.

Isn't it worth it?

RECOMMENDED FURTHER READING:

"Secrets of Health and Beauty," Linda Clark, 1970, Devin-Adair Company.

"Stay Young Longer," Linda Clark, 1968, Devin-Adair Company.

"Let's Get Well," Adelle Davis, 1965, Harcourt, Brace & World, Inc.

"Feel Like a Million," Catharyn Elwood, 1965, Devin-Adair Company.

"Foods For Glamour," Jack La Lanne, 1961, Prentice Hall, Inc.

"Food Combining Made Easy," Dr. Herbert M. Shelton, 1964, Dr. Shelton's Health School, San Antonio, Texas.

"East, Drink and Be Healthy," Agnes Toms, 1968, Devin-Adair Company.

CHAPTER THREE

WHAT YOUR BODY *GETS* FOR NOURISHMENT

1. *The Insufficiency of Modern Diets*

We have seen how vitamins, minerals, proteins, amino acids, and enzymes all interact with one another, and how all are essential to keep the organs of the body acting in harmony and to keep you feeling young and alive. We've seen how you can't pick and choose among them; they are a team.

Now let's see how many of them can be found in our everyday selection of foods; the things we eat on the spur of the moment or from force of habit—especially things we grab at a coffee shop for breakfast or lunch, almost without thinking.

Let's consider things that are on the coffee wagon at the office or available in cafeterias and coffee shops in schools, office buildings and sporting events. Let's look at them for the amount of *nutrition* they do or don't provide. Then we'll look into what we get *instead* of nutrition in these few sample foods.

BREAKFAST:

Cold cereal—Most vitamins have been processed out and replaced by artificial ones; in both the milk and the cereal. The sugar contains no nourishment either.

Scrambled eggs—While the eggs may have had some nourishment to begin with, they have been smothered with grease or fat from the frying process. The toast will be from de-vitalized white bread, no doubt, and covered with butter and super-sweet jelly.

Pancakes—Made from bland white flour, fried on a greasy griddle, covered with butter (more fat) and soaked with sweetened (artificially) syrup.

Donuts—Made from white flour again, fried in grease again. If it's a plain donut, it's a mouthful of nothing. More likely it's covered with refined white sugar (valueless) or chocolate or possibly filled with artificially sweetened jelly.

Coffee—Valueless as nutrition. The sugar and cream pose their own problems.

COFFEE BREAK:

Danish pastry—Made from white flour with no nutrients left and thus no nourishment. Often covered with sugar or filled with a sweet-tasting cream.

Coffee—See above.

Donut—See above.

LUNCH:

Bacon & Tomato—Probably on white bread (again), possibly toasted and buttered. The lettuce will be wilted and was probably sprayed while growing, and the tomatoes have probably been given an additive to grow bigger or to look redder.

Tuna salad—Aside from the white bread and the presence of mercury in the fish, this might still do you some good.

Hamburger—In the better shops the meat may actually still have some value, but that bun is made from valueless white flour again and will just fill you up with empty calories.

French Fries—You lost a lot of the potato's value when the skin was removed and now it's all covered with grease. Maybe there's value left in the catsup—unless it's lost in the chemicals used to thicken it and color it.

Spaghetti—Nothing here but starch and salt. The tomato sauce may have a little value but again it may also be chemically treated. Nourishment probably lies only in the cheese!

Apple pie—The crust is made from white flour, the apples were not considered good enough for sale as eating apples and have been drenched in artificially sweetened syrup—after removal of the skins which contain whatever nutrition might have been obtained. Now bury it under over-sweetened and artificially flavored ice cream, which seldom contains cream anymore.

Chocolate cake—More empty calories, since it's made from white flour and artificial sweeteners, shortening and coloring.

AFTERNOON SNACK:

Coke—No nourishment whatever, but plenty of sugar.

Malted milk—Probably some benefit left in the malt, but oh that sweetened chocolate and the ice cream!

Pizza—White flour again; full of oil; but maybe that tomato sauce saves it. But that's doubtful since cost-cutting is the name of the game in this business; what chance have real tomatoes against chemicals?

Hot dog—The less said about frankfurter meat (whatever isn't actually cereal or coloring) the better. Maybe a smidgen of nourishment survives in the mustard or sauerkraut. I doubt it.

Hopefully the mythical American who eats the above very regularly (and didn't most of us during high school?) will exercise a little more imagination on the supper meal and get some nourishment in spite of himself (or herself).

Every year the United States leads the world in food production and in food consumption. Yet we are plagued with the same diseases and afflictions as the rest of the civilized world. Something must be wrong.

Millions of pairs of glasses are sold every year in the United States. Poor eyesight is improved by vitamin A in the diet. As we have seen, vitamin A is found in such widely-consumed things as spinach, carrots, liver, eggs and tomatoes. Why then do so many Americans suffer from poor eyesight?

The same thing could be said for skin blemishes. The cosmetic and drug industries make millions of dollars a year selling creams and lotions to hide or "cure" skin blemishes. Vitamin A is usually the deficiency when that occurs. Since we grow and consume so many popular things containing that vitamin, why should the problem still be big enough to support an industry?

Every year businesses are plagued with employee absences due to the common cold. Colds are usually prevented and combatted by vitamins A and C, which are present in spinach, asparagus, oranges, sweet potatoes and tomatoes. We produce plenty of these foods, so why should there be a problem? If these vitamins were only found in rare foods, or little-known herbs, it might be understandable.

Insomnia is indicative of a lack of vitamin B-complex and the amnio acid valine. Both valine and vitamin B are found in milk and peanuts. So why are drug firms so successful in selling pills to put people to sleep who can't seem to fall asleep?

Tooth decay. How many cavities a year are filled by American dentists? How many false teeth are sold to replace those that fall out or must be extracted? Yet the proper intake of vitamins B and

D, together with calcium, should prevent this. Where are all three found—in milk! If we consume over 70 billion quarts of milk a year, how can it be that we have so many cavities?

The wig industry is very big business in this country. Hairpieces for bald spots and wigs for the whole head are sold by the tens of thousands. Thousands of other bald and partially bald people do nothing about their hair. People with thinning hair buy all manner of lotions and tonics to retard the loss of their hair. Yet we know that the best thing for it is vitamin B and the amino acid methionine. Where are both of those ingredients found? Eggs. With 60,000,000,000 eggs produced every year in this country, it does seem rather unusual that there is so much baldness.

Perhaps the answer lies in understanding something that happened in Guatemala in 1960.

In order to combat the malnutrition of 50 particularly sickly Guatemalan children, an American scientist working there duplicated the composition of the chicken feed that he used to feed his chickens back in New Jersey. He fed them on this diet of "chicken feed" for eight weeks instead of their accustomed poor diet which had been barely keeping them alive; alive but very sickly. During those eight weeks the children all put on weight, lost sores and swellings, and took a renewed interest in life.

What's the point? Simply to indicate that there can be more genuine nutrition in the daily diet of American chickens than in the Guatemalan's overly-starched, poverty-level diet.

Americans put more care and expertise into determining what their chickens, dogs, horses and sheep will eat than they do into what they themselves must. They know that animals are healthier (and sell for higher prices) and produce healthier eggs or wool, or race faster, if they eat certain vitamins and minerals. It never seems to occur to us that if *we* wish to be healthy and remain free from disease and discomfort, we too must eat the correct diet rather than any old thing that pleases our sweet tooth, our sense of smell, or our eyes.

2. Causes of Poor Health

According to respected doctors, the six principal causes of disease, in order of importance, are:

1. Emotional upset.
2. Nutritional deficiency.
3. Poisons ingested.
4. Infections.
5. Accidents.
6. Inherited diseases.

In this book, we are concerned with 2 and 3, but it should be noted how far down the list are things like catching an infection or inheriting a disease. We were not meant by nature to be ill or ugly due to poor health. Four of the six principal causes are from things we (personally, or via our society) bring upon ourselves.

Nature has set up a master plan for perfect health. If we adhere to it we thrive; if we don't, we deteriorate. There's nothing magical about it, nor any element of capricious chance. If we play by the rules we win; if we don't, we suffer the consequences—old age and illness.

The problem is that so much of society has forgotten the rules for so long, and gone off on a self-indulgent binge of eating things that look good, or satisfy their sweet tooth, or maybe just things that everybody else eats (no matter whether they are nourishing), that it becomes increasingly difficult for the one who comes to his or her senses to be able to get back to living by the rules.

We were meant to eat the pure, whole food which nature provided. We were meant to breathe pure air and drink pure water. When we tamper with nature, bypass it or try to outsmart it, we are going to run into difficulties. That's one of the rules.

The repair materials which nature provided to keep our bodies functioning in top form, and which should be in every diet, are no longer there in sufficient amounts to keep us healthy.

Our bodies have 60 or more elements and each has its job to perform. If any of them are missing, or not on the job 100 percent of the time, trouble will develop sooner or later. The thing to remember is that all 60 are needed; 30 or 15 will not be able to do the job.

If, for instance, you are not getting enough calcium in your diet, your body will "steal" it from other areas in the body where it is stored—eventually causing a breakdown somewhere. Irritability, arthritis, osteoporosis of the bones, or even tooth decay may develop. And calcium is merely one element. The more elements that are in insufficient supply, the more problems you will have, and the sooner they will develop.

Infectious diseases caused by a germ or virus can be more serious if protective elements are lacking in the body and its resistance is lowered. Every day millions of cells wear out, get damaged or destroyed. Every day your body tries to replace, rebuild and repair them to maintain health and prevent disease. The only way you get those materials is from your diet.

The problem is that we eat what we *like* rather than what we need. If we would at least eat both we might be better off except that much of what we like is harmful rather than neutral for the body.

Two thirds of the human race suffers from a deficient diet. Their daily diet lacks energy, protective values and tissue-repairing factors. We fill ourselves up with empty calories which do nothing to *build* us up. This leads to a single deficiency and then to multiple ones, and finally to "old age" diseases.

Very few people in this country sit down to a meal having anything like the nutrition in a can of dog food.

Afflictions like a cleft palate, weak heart, poor vision, poor hearing, sub-normal gland activity have all been traced to nutrient-deficiencies in the mother. The birth defects revealed in the thalidomide scandal, originally blamed on the drug, were found to be the result of a lack of vitamin B2 in the mothers' diet. The drug only complicated the situation.

3. *The Harmfulness of Modern Diets*

If it were just a question of eating the wrong foods, foods that have no value in them, perhaps the answer would lie in eliminating them from one's diet and substituting more nourishing foods. A hundred years ago this might have been the simple answer. However, food production, transportation, processing, and distribution has changed radically in that time and all have had a hand in determining the food value of fruits, vegetables, meats, fish and dairy products. Most people in this country are not aware of the enormous impact of these changes upon those food values.

CHEMICAL ADDITIVES

Recently, investigators for the Food & Drug Administration tested 25 meals at different public eating places. At each place they found DDT in the meat, potatoes, pie and coffee with cream. Researchers have concluded from this and other tests that few if any foods today are entirely free from DDT.

This is quite shocking when you consider that DDT was only invented in 1939 and did not reach widespread use until the middle of the 1940's—a little over a quarter of a century ago.

Where does it all come from? It is initially sprayed onto plants and trees to control insects. Sometimes the rain washes the residue into streams and rivers, contaminating fish. Sometimes it is sprayed on large areas from the air and the winds carry it to areas not intended for its use (like cattle-grazing land) and it is ingested by animals which are later eaten by humans or whose products (milk and eggs etc.) are eaten. It is a very persistent chemical and is spreading across the globe and through the seas.

Is it really needed in the first place? If you believe that faulty farming methods should be excused by cover-up devices, regardless of the ecological and nutritional consequences, perhaps you will accept DDT as just one of the hazards of modern living.

Erosion robs the topsoil of our farmlands. One cause of erosion is non-rotational farming: growing the same product in the same plot of ground year in and year out. We have all learned in school how this depletes the soil of certain chemicals after a few years, leading to erosion, and that planting different crops in a given field each year renews and replenishes the soil.

A sick soil will produce sick and weakened plants which are more susceptible to disease and insect attack. Plants which are properly nourished with minerals are disease-resistant and can be grown without pesticide sprays. It is the plant that is deficient in minerals which becomes infested with pests. We call them "pests," but they are really part of nature's plan for keeping up the ecological balance.

In a purely natural state, an acorn grows into an oak tree, sheds more acorns to grow into more trees, and eventually will die and fall to earth, where it will slowly decompose back into the soil from which it came. This is an example of the ecological balance.

So, also, with farm products. Under nature's plan, corn (for instance) would grow by feeding on certain minerals in the soil, blossoming into fine yellow ears. The ears would eventually rot and return to the earth to re-enrich the soil during the winter and then repeat the cycle.

When man discovered that corn was good to eat, he carried off the corn. He carried it to his home—not very far from the field in those days—and ate it. The cobs were discarded and found their way back into the earth—not necessarily in the same field from which they came, but the cycle was nevertheless complete.

Insects were nature's way of seeing to it that a certain amount of the corn was not carried away, but was plowed under right there in the field.

As long as man ate only what he needed and left the rest to rot in the field or to be eaten by insects, the balance in nature was preserved. But when an entire farm would be devoted to the growing of corn, and expensive mechanical equipment was invested in (in order to reduce the costs of feeding and paying for large harvesting crews), the goal of increased production dictated that as little corn as possible be allowed to spoil. Enter insect sprays.

So now the new vicious cycle becomes apparent:

- Super fertilizers are employed to increase production.
- Insecticides are used to limit spoilage.
- The soil is impoverished by loss of the product.
- The impoverished soil produces diseased plants.
- Diseased plants attract a hardier breed of insects.
- New chemicals are used on the new pests.
- Pests develop immunity to the chemicals.
- *Stronger* chemicals are devised!

The final element in the equation is that thanks to modern plumbing and garbage disposal systems, the minerals in that corn cob are lost forever to the soil; the garbage is treated and the human waste is treated before they return to earth.

So DDT and a host of other pesticides and insecticides have

been used in the never-ending quest to keep ahead of the evolution of the insect world. And we are ingesting this strong chemical in all kinds of food. We are storing it in our fat tissues. Apologists for the pesticide industry tell us that the amounts we are getting are nowhere near lethal doses.

First of all, they cannot really measure what are "the amounts we are getting" because they do not even know all the different meats, fruits and vegetables we are ingesting DDT in. Second, due to its persistence in the soil and in fat tissues, we are being poisoned on the installment plan rather than flat-out.

When people die of "cancer," "heart disease" and "pneumonia" and autopsies indicate large accumulations of DDT in the body, it is a reasonable question to ask what role DDT may have played. And the person seriously interested in nutrition can only read in trepidation that a new chemical called "chlordane," reportedly five times as deadly as DDT, is gaining in popularity.

But the inclusion of DDT in our diet is an "accident;" it was not intended that way. We are just going to have to live with it and try to avoid the effects of its contamination. There are other things added to our foods intentionally. There are things like additives, flavor enhancers, preservatives, coloring agents, and even anti-biotics.

Many kinds of *fish,* especially deep sea fish, are treated with chlortetracycline as an anti-biotic. We are told that boiling the fish will remove all traces of the chemical. What we are not told is that it would take 30 minutes of boiling to do the job completely. Such long cooking isn't noted for enhancing the flavor of fish. As a matter of fact it would destroy the food value.

It is also not often that people boil fish. Usually they broil or fry it. The results of broiling are unclear, but frying does not elim-inate all traces of the anti-biotic (and that is according to the A.M.A).

Most *eggs* consumed by Americans are infertile. Stores pay more for them because they keep longer on the shelf (or the re-frigerator section, if you prefer). These infertile eggs lack vita-min E.

Weedicides are used on *Fruits* and *Vegetables* to reduce the labor costs of weeding the truck gardens. Hormones are injected in fruits to make them grow larger. Sweet potatoes are injected with a reddish dye. White potatoes receive an anti-sprouting additive. Cucumbers and turnips may be dipped in paraffin for longer shelf-life.

Lemons are washed in a chemical dip to reduce tip-end decay. Grapes are treated to prevent mold. Canned fruits are put through a chemical dip to remove their skins. Asparagus is washed with a mold inhibitor. Nuts are bleached for uniformity of color.

Additives are added to many *Baking Products* in order to cut down on the necessity for using eggs. Bread receives artificial chemicals to keep it "soft" and "fresh-feeling."

Milk gets pasteurized and homogenized, a process which decreases enzymes, minerals and vitamins contained in it. Artificial vitamins are then added.

Farm Animal Feeds now commonly contain anti-biotics and hormones. Their fat tissues fill up (with water) making them more valuable on the auction block—but no more nourishing.

Grains are milled and then bleached, which eliminates any mineral traces that survived the milling. Vitamin E is one of the casualties; it was intended by nature to mend and strengthen heart muscles. Someone dies of heart disease every two minutes in the United States. Diseases of the heart and blood vessels cause more than twice the deaths from cancer.

Brown rice is polished and refined and loses B vitamins, proteins and minerals in the process. Green citrus fruits are picked early and then dyed to look appetizing. Some of the dyes have been proven to be poisonous and cancer-producing.

There are nearly 3,000 chemicals which are permitted to be added to foods or to come in contact with them. About a thousand of them are things used in place of eggs, fats and other nourishment; 650 are synthetic flavorings to replace real nuts, fruit, butter and herb flavorings. The remaining 1,300 are used to give false freshness and false texture, and to permit long shelf-life.

What a price our civilization pays for the so-called "high standard of living" we talk about so much! Why does under-nourishment on the one hand, and installment-plan-poisoning on the other have to be the price we pay? And how are you ever going to look your glamorous best without the natural nutrition and *with* all the unnatural?

THE DE-VITALIZATION OF MILK

Milk is 87 percent water, so it is not by any means a concentrated food. Yet it is a rich food—in its natural state. The amount of protein, minerals, vitamins and enzymes it contains depends on the diet and health of the cow—something you have no way of knowing.

When it gets to the processing plants, pasteurizing destroys the vitamin C and enzymes; homogenizing destroys the cellular structure. The artificial vitamins used at the plant to "fortify" it are weak sisters indeed to the ones that were removed or killed. Just to complicate things more, if it is bottled in glass and left on your doorstep on a sunny day for a few hours, the sunlight will destroy the vitamin B2.

It is estimated that 25 percent of the natural vitamin C and 38 percent of the B-Complex are destroyed in the pasteurizing. This process, intended to kill disease-causing germs, also kills an enzyme called phosphatase. Without this enzyme, the body does not absorb calcium and phosphate from the milk. Yet the very test for determining the success of pasteurization is whether the phosphatase is dead!

Maybe this is a clue to why we can consume so much "milk" in this country and still keep all those dentists busy. . . .

According to a report in the American Journal of Obstetrics and Gynecology, May 1935, pasteurizing was introduced in Berlin in 1904. The incidence of cases of scurvy rose dramatically about the same time. An investigation was made as to the cause and the pasteurization was discontinued. The number of cases of scurvy declined just as dramatically and as suddenly as they had increased.

It would seem clear that the big dairies in this country choose to pasteurize milk because it helps their problem of long distance distribution rather than for any health reasons. After all, if health were the criterion, why would they continue to de-vitalize the milk? Why wouldn't they seek other ways of controlling the entry of bacteria into the milk? Such as, perhaps, greater control over the diet and milking procedures of the cows and the workers who come in contact with the milk and its containers?

THE DE-VITALIZING OF BREAD AND FLOUR

In ancient times, and all the way down to comparatively recent times, wheat was crushed between two stones—"millstones." This process crushed the wheat kernels enough for humans to eat and still preserved all parts of the kernel, the part that is today called "wheat germ."

When it is ground up fine it is called flour; if coarsely ground, cereal. The value of stone-grinding is that the grain is ground very slowly and remains unheated.

Just over 100 years ago, in 1870 a steel roller mill was invented which replaced stone-milling. This machine ground wheat into flour one hundred times faster and therefore not only increased the speed of the operation, it increased the capability of the mill to handle much more wheat if the farmers would grow it.

But the flour so produced was a nutritionally weaker flour because the heat generated by the roller mill greatly reduced the protein content, destroyed the structure of the wheat, and caused the delicate wheat germ to gum up the roller.

In the interests of smoother production, removal of the wheat germ was added to the milling operation. An extra benefit to the millers was that without the wheat germ the flour kept much longer before turning rancid. Production rose, sales rose, and profits rose.

However, the incidence of heart disease also began to rise around this time. Today we know that the missing wheat germ is rich in vitamin E, which is vital to the heart's blood vessels.

As long ago as 1946 the Minnesota Experimental Agriculture Station reported that cattle, deprived of vitamin E after seeming to be in perfect health, suddenly dropped dead of heart disease. When the wheat germ was restored to their feed the deaths from heart disease stopped.

But they didn't stop with the removal of vitamin E from the flour. Around the turn of the century we began "bleaching" flour in order to "age" it more rapidly and to give it a whiter, "purer" look. In the 1940's the FDA finally forbade the use of a bleach called Agene because research had shown it caused running fits and mental deterioration in test dogs.

Today flours are bleached with oxides of nitrogen, chlorine,

nitrosyl chloride, chlorine dioxide and benzoyl peroxide mixed
with chemical salts.

Should you remain unconvinced of the debilitating effects for
our nutrition resulting from the milling of white flour, here is an
analysis of the vitamin and mineral losses made by the University
of California College of Agriculture published in 1960:

Thiamin	about 80% lost
Riboflavin	60%
Niacin	75%
Pantothenic Acid	50%
Pyridoxine	50%
Calcium	50%
Phosphorus	70%
Iron	80%
Manganese	98%
Magnesium	75%
Potassium	50%
Copper	65%

You will note when shopping that most bread is labelled "enriched" so, you ask, how can it be so nutritionally empty if it is
labelled "enriched?" The same way milk is called "fortified" after
natural vitamins and minerals are removed by the processing.

In 1941 a National Nutrition Conference was called in Wash-
ington. It was at this conference that flour millers were permitted
to "enrich" the bread by adding artificial vitamins and minerals
(not, however, vitamin E). But our whole approach to natural nutrition for natural beauty and health is that if the food is so bad
that it has to be "enriched" or "fortified" it should be rejected!

Some other countries are taking positive steps along this direction. Canada has passed a law prohibiting the enrichment of bread
via synthetic vitamins. If a bread is to be sold as high-vitamin
bread it must be the original vitamins found in the wheat, not
imitations.

Switzerland taxes white bread. The tax is distributed to the
makers of whole wheat bread to help bring down their prices so
that more people can afford it.

4. *Special Problem of Sugar vs. Teeth*

Nutritionists realize that the condition of the teeth is a reliable indication of the condition of the bony structures, organs and tissues of our bodies. Poor cleaning of the teeth contributes to tooth decay but it is not the sole reason, perhaps not even the prime one. Decay also reaches the teeth from the flow of blood reaching the pulp of the tooth. Blood that is not carrying vitamins A, B, and D, calcium and phosphorus is not properly nourishing the teeth from the inside and decay will result.

Dental decay is the most prevalent disease known to mankind. At least 98 percent of the population in this country suffers from some degree of dental decay. It is the informed opinion of many dentists and nutritionists that *sound nutrition* is the best method of combatting dental decay and the destruction of supporting bone structures. And surprising as it may seem to you, where dentists and nutritionists have been able to obtain the full cooperation of patients, they have been successful in controlling dental disease. Catharyn Elwood speaks of a dentist who practiced dentistry in Los Angeles for 35 years *without a dentist's chair!* He cared for people's teeth via controlling their diet. And you can, too.

Since 1850 American consumption of sugar has climbed from 10 lbs. per person annually to about 100 pounds per person. Many researchers have detected a related rise in tooth decay in the same period. Leading dental authorities concur in the assertion that the most destructive decay agents acting upon the outside of teeth are the bacteria which thrive on refined white sugar, creating acids. These acids, in turn, attack the tooth enamel and create or help to create cavities.

Cola and carbonated drinks contain phosphoric acid, which has been shown to produce etching of teeth enamel, thus rendering the tooth more susceptible to attack by harmful acids in the mouth.

So, some good rules to follow in fighting cavities would be the following:

- Brush teeth within 5 minutes of the end of every meal.

- Eat generous amounts of green and yellow vegetables.

- Supplement them with vitamin A from fish liver oil capsules.

- Avoid refined foods (white sugar and white flour products).

- Increase your intake of foods rich in the B-complex vitamins, such as liver, brewer's yeast, and wheat germ.

The B-vitamins help prevent tooth decay. A lack of Pantothenic Acid (one of the B-Family) causes teeth to decay rapidly. Yet, in order to burn sugar, B-vitamins must be borrowed from the remainder of the diet—which rarely has enough for its own calories.

In a controlled experiment in a large clinic, a diet of meat, fish, eggs, fresh fruits and vegetables was given, *plus* sugary desserts. The addition of the desserts caused conditions close to that of a nervous breakdown. Despite the otherwise good diet, the sugar was robbing vitamin B1 from their bodies.

Refined sugar is found primarily in white sugar and in commercial glucose. Unrefined sugar will be found in honey, maple sugar, fruit sugars, molasses and sorghum.

Sugar content of some common fruits and vegetables:

3%—Asparagus, brussels sprouts, celery, cucumbers, eggplant, kale, lettuce, rhubarb, spinach, squash.

5%—Beets, cabbage, cauliflower, onions, green peppers, pumpkin, radishes, green beans, water cress.

7%—Avocado, grapefruit, lemon, loganberries, olives, strawberries, watermelon.

10%—Blackberries, cantaloupe, cranberries, oranges, peaches, pineapple, raspberries, carrots, turnips.

15%—Apples, apricots, cherries, grapes, nectarines, pears, pineapple, lima beans, peas, corn, sweet potatoes, navy beans, brown rice (cooked).

20%—Bananas, figs, plums, prunes.

25%—Dried apples, dried apricots, dried figs, dried prunes, raisins.

Pyorrhea is another dental problem to be concerned about. This is the wasting away of the bone foundation of the teeth due to a lack of vitamin C. It usually does not come until after age 40.

The walls break down due to a lack of the cement structure furnished by vitamin C, and soon the gums begin to recede.

We have all seen how unsightly people look who have this disease; their teeth appear to be growing out of their gums, with only the tip of the root still covered. Actually the exact reverse is happening: the gums are receding from the teeth, leaving more and more of the root visible. Proper amounts of vitamin C in the person's diet would have prevented this, and can still arrest it.

Sugar is not a necessary article of diet, nor is it a food essential (neither is refined flour). Sugar is a concentrated carbohydrate containing no vitamins or minerals of any kind. Even if you consume no sugar at all, your body will convert 68 percent of the other foods in your diet into sugar, so the intake of refined white sugar and artificial sweeteners is superfluous.

If you feel you can't get along without satisfying your sweet tooth, you can get natural sugar from fruits and you could also try sweetening things with honey.

A word about commercial glucose. This is used as a filler in such products as canned fruit, candy, jams, jellies, preserves, cheese spreads, frozen fruits, ice cream and soft drinks. It is a subtle sweetener and just because it isn't obviously sweet, it is possible to consume large amounts without being aware of it. Read labels! This is a very widespread ingredient. Yet it was linked to one type of diabetes in animals as long ago as 1948.

Canada banned glucose in soft drinks.

Remember that sugar, like alcohol and tobacco, can be habit-forming. Although it has been found that the more sugar you take the more you crave, fortunately it is conversely true that the less you take the less you crave!

If you have a sweet tooth it is preferable to get your sweetness in dark molasses (unsulphured) and honey since they possess the same vitamins and minerals. Yet they are all still dangerously concentrated sweets. Better to gradually eliminate your craving!

RECOMMENDED FURTHER READING:

"Secrets of Health and Beauty," Linda Clark, 1970, Devin-Adair Company.

"Stay Young Longer," Linda Clark, 1968, Devin-Adair Company.

"Let's Get Well," Adelle Davis, 1965, Harcourt, Brace & World, Inc.

"Feel Like a Million," Catharyn Elwood, 1965, Devin-Adair Company.

"Foods For Glamour," Jack La Lanne, 1961, Prentice-Hall, Inc.

"Food Combining Made Easy," Dr. Herbert M. Shelton, 1964, Dr. Shelton's Health School, San Antonio, Texas.

"Eat, Drink and Be Healthy," Agnes Toms, 1968, Devin-Adair Company.

"Vitamin E; Your Key to A Healthy Heart," Herbert Bailey, 1964, ARC Books, Inc.

CHAPTER FOUR

BEAUTY FROM WITHIN—VIA PROPER NUTRITION

Being overweight is just as much a symptom of *mal*nutrition as being underweight. Let's repeat that again so that it will be impressed upon you: PEOPLE WHO ARE OVERWEIGHT ARE SUFFERING FROM MALNUTRITION.

We tend to think of malnutrition in terms of starving refugees in Asia, but when "malnutrition" is translated into its two parts, it is easily seen that it is not limited to under-nourished; it only means "bad nutrition"—not getting the *right* foods.

A handy list of foods to avoid:

Refined white sugar products:

- Syrups, candy, jam, jelly, marmalade, ice cream, soft drinks, chewing gum.

Refined white flour products:

- White bread, noodles, macaroni, spaghetti, cakes, pies, cookies, rolls, doughnuts.

Packaged breakfast foods (especially the sugared ones!)

Canned fruits (in syrup).

Canned vegetables (salt and sugar added).

Hot and irritating condiments:
- Strong vinegar, hot sauces, red pepper.

Stimulants and depressants:
- Coffee, tea, chocolate, colas, alcohol, tobacco.

Canned, pasteurized and condensed milk.

You say you can't possibly do without *all* of those everyday things? Choose your poison. Which of them are you so dearly attached to that you will sacrifice your health for? Before you make this awesome decision, let us consider what foods you *ought* to eat as substitutes for the above. Give yourself half a chance and you can become as attached to many of the good foods as you are to the bad. The human body is amazingly adaptive!

WHAT ABOUT FATS AND CHOLESTEROL?

Beautiful skin, radiant health, and calm nerves are impossible without the *proper* fats in your diet. Fats combine with phosphorus to form part of every cell in the body.

Even when we avoid cholesterol-rich foods, the body still manufactures it. Your body needs cholesterol in order to manufacture the sex hormones, bile, and vitamin D. So the problem is not to *eliminate* fats from the diet, but to eat the correct kind and amount.

So don't deny yourself cholesterol-rich foods. Rather, try eating foods rich in *lecithin*. Lecithin is often called "Nature's Jailer" because it imprisons certain substances and releases others. It is an essential part of all animal and vegetable cells, and turns up in abundance in the heart, kidney, liver, brain and endocrine glands. It prevents liver and artery degeneration, by holding fats in solution instead of allowing them to accumulate on the walls of arteries and throughout the liver.

Lecithin also prevents fatigue due to nerve-sheath destruction. Without lecithin, the nerves become tense, on edge and raw. More to the point of this book, lecithin prevents many skin problems.

SELECTING A NATURAL BEAUTY DIET

Ideally you should check with a nutritional physician before starting any diet. Since they are in such scant supply in this country, see your own doctor frequently during the course of the diet.

One of the first things to remember is that it's your *entire* food intake which you must watch, not just the three meals. You must watch out for the frills that you find around the house, around the office, or in the restaurant, that can cancel out any benefit you derive from your controlled diet.

You will be smart enough to ignore the pretzels, crackers, and potato chips at a party, but don't forget to pass up things like chewing gum and after-dinner mints. Ordering a baked potato at a restaurant instead of mashed or fried is useless if you let the waiter pour sour cream or gobs of butter on it. The same would go for the mayonnaise on a chicken salad sandwich or butter sauce on peas.

It is also important to be dieting at the right time—or at least not to be dieting at the *wrong* time. You should not start a diet during times of stress. If you are worrying over money, over domestic affairs, or over having just lost a job, that's enough of a strain on your nervous system.

If constipation occurs during your diet, it may be a sign that the poisons, after being dislodged, are being distributed throughout your body prior to elimination. Many doctors will prescribe large doses of vitamin C to neutralize the poisons.

When you return to solid foods after your de-toxifying diet, the best advice is to begin gently. Choose foods that are easily digested in small amounts, and chew them thoroughly.

DE-TOXIFYING YOURSELF

The first step in dieting for overall health—as opposed to dieting merely to lose weight—is to de-toxify your body. As an ordinary, average American woman, your body is clogged with poisons, drugs, preservatives, alkalizers, acidifiers, artificial sweeteners, artificial softeners, animal hormones, chemical dyes, antioxidants, hydrogenators, *ad nauseam*—pun intended!

All of these things are abnormal to the human body and must be neutralized or excreted, otherwise disease can result, or even death in some cases. A de-toxifying diet is needed to cleanse the insides of your body and to remove this "debris" from your organs, glands, tissues and blood stream.

It is particularly important to clean the walls of the small intestine which has become incrusted with undigested food. This "debris" forms a barrier to the proper absorption of important nutrients into the bloodstream.

Try this de-toxifying diet for ten days:

- The juice of 2½ lemons (2 tablespoonsful).
- 2 tablespoons of black strap molasses.

Mix them in an 8 oz. glass of medium hot water and drink it six to 12 times a day.

If you can, repeat it 3 or 4 times a year. This high vitamin-mineral cleansing diet will help you to look and feel at your best. It will dissolve and eliminate toxins and waste anywhere in the body. It will give your digestive system a rest and purify the glands, cells and bloodstream. It often assists in the loss of a pound a day, also. It is recommended by Stanley A. Burroughs, a teacher of Natural Health.

Another possibility for a de-toxifying diet is as follows:

- Fresh organic carrot juice (from your own juicer).
  - or
- Well-washed, well-chewed grapes.
  - or
- Whole grapefruit and celery.

Try that one for three days and then for the next three weeks confine yourself to raw fruits and vegetables (uncooked). The vegetables can be used in a tasty salad with a dressing made of cold-pressed oils, apple cider vinegar, or lemon juice. You might season the vegetables with "seasalt" which contains more minerals than table salt but tastes the same. Fruits can be made into salads, fruit cups or eaten separately.

You must beware of the alternative of complete fasting. When we use that term we mean no food or drink except plain water. If you do this, you are forcing the body to feed on itself. Thus you are providing your body with an undiluted menu of poisons. The reason is that the fatty tissues, where the insecticides and other poisons have stored themselves, begin to break down and these poisons are rapidly released into the bloodstream. Without half trying, you can literally poison yourself!

Alternatively, the intake of fresh juices and raw fruits and vegetables will release the poisons slowly and not suddenly. They will be diluted and the tissues will have other foods to feed on.

After de-toxification, avoid refined, processed and additived food of any kind. If the health food store near you does not stock organically-grown fruits and vegetables (raised by farmers who do not spray them with chemicals) perhaps they may recommend a source you could purchase them from. The degree of inconvenience you are willing to go to in order to remain healthy and improve the natural way is a good indicator of how serious you are about rejuvenating yourself.

FOODS TO AVOID AFTER DE-TOXIFYING

Years ago (generations ago, really) everyone automatically was eating pure, uncontaminated food because that was all there was. Today we must search for such hard-to-find food as raw vegetables (organically-grown) and pay extra for it. The informed shopper searching in the supermarket for plain, unadulterated, nourishing food has been compared to Diogenes searching in vain for the honest man.

In addition to the list provided a few pages back of foods to avoid, one should exercise great care in selecting *meats*. Something like 80-85 percent of the meat in this country comes from animals that were fed stilbestrol in their feed. This is a synthetic hormone which was given them to add weight in the form of fat and water.

Stilbestrol has been found to produce cancer in mice, minks and rats just from eating scraps of meat from animals (cattle and chickens) that had been fed stilbestrol.

Chickens are also often dipped in aureomycin, an antibiotic, to prevent spoilage. Chickens so dipped will last two to three weeks instead of one week. Such chickens are supposed to be labelled "Acronized," and cooking is supposed to eliminate the antibiotic.

FOODS TO SEEK OUT

The key to good health is to seek out food that is *whole,* that has suffered the least amount of tampering. Nature does provide the proper balance of food factors. When we remove one factor, the effectiveness of that food will be quite different than in its natural state.

We should remember that before fire was harnessed, man ate his food raw. There might be a moral in the fact that when zoos started serving cooked food to their animals, the animals started to exhibit the same diseases as man. Zoos have reverted to feeding raw food for some time.

In the early 1940's an experiment was conducted on two groups of cats. One group was fed raw milk and raw meat and the others were fed cooked food and pasteurized milk. The first group of cats stayed healthy and produced healthy kittens for several observed generations.

The second group soon displayed many ailments of our modern society: gingivitis, loss of teeth, loss of fertility, labor difficulties, irritability, diminished interest, allergies, infections, diarrhea, pneumonia, heart trouble, kidney disease, thyroid disease, etc.

However, healthful eating can still be pleasant eating. It just takes more imagination. Your friends and associates may not have the courage to embark on this health plan, but you should not give in to their entreaties to make exceptions to your diet just for them. There are ways of not inconveniencing them.

For instance, you can go to friends' houses for the evening— after dinner hour. At your own home, get them to try some of your diet and provide other things which they may be more used to. At their house for dinner all you can do is select among what they serve the lesser of the various evils. Apologize for not taking more by pleading "small appetite," "late lunch," "on a diet," or "I never take coffee this late—it keeps me awake."

A little dry wine with a meal is good. Wine has some nutritional value due to its B vitamins, as well as potassium, magnesium, sodium, calcium, iron and phosphorus. In addition to nourishment, dry wine stimulates the digestion. But only take 3 ounces and only before or during the meal. Before the meal it stimulates appetite and during the meal helps you to assimilate the food.

WONDER FOODS

Do I really have to spend the better part of a day in the store reading labels to see what nourishment I'm getting? Do I really have to drive to the country every few days to buy fresh fruits and vegetables? Isn't there an easier way to get the proper nourishment? Yes there is if you have a health store nearby. That's where you'll find those things Nutritionists call the "Wonder Foods:"

- Blackstrap molasses.

- Wheat germ.

- Brewer's yeast.

- Yogurt.
- Lecithin.
- Liver.

They are called "wonder foods" because, ounce for ounce, they contain more repair materials than any other foods. Each is loaded with vitamins and minerals and together they give you 13 different vitamins and 17 minerals! If you didn't mind the monotony, you might exist on these six foods alone.

BLACKSTRAP MOLASSES

Blackstrap molasses is one of the foods richest in iron—there being enough in one tablespoonful to equal that in nine eggs. It is a good laxative; stops falling hair; contains more calcium than milk; can be used in cooking, added to yogurt, in hot water as a "tea," or in milk as a "shake."

Blackstrap molasses contains:

Calcium.
Phosphorus.
Iron.
Copper.
Potassium.
B-vitamins (7 of them).

WHEAT GERM

Wheat germ is the embryo of the seed which nature intended to become next year's wheat crop. It is milled out of our wheat. We have also noted that the wheat thereby loses its vitamin E. Well this is an excellent way to get it back. In addition, half a cup of wheat germ contains 4 eggs' worth of protein (24 grams). It can be added into baking without altering the flavor and is therefore useful in biscuits, muffins, breads, waffles, pancakes and meat loaves.

Wheat germ contains:

Vitamin B1.	Vitamin B6.
Vitamin B2.	Vitamin E.

Proteins.   Iron.
Copper.   Manganese.

BREWER'S YEAST

One of the best and cheapest sources of vitamin B. Yeast has, of course, been in use since the time of the Romans. *Brewer's* yeast is a by-product of the brewing of beer. It helps to lower the cholesterol level; helps control cirrhosis of the liver; and helps clear up acne.

Brewer's yeast contains:

Vitamins	*Minerals*	
B1	Phosphorus	Sodium
B2	Potassium	Iron
B6	Magnesium	Tin
Niacin	Silicon	Boron
Choline	Calcium	Gold
Inositol	Copper	Silver
Pantothenic acid	Manganese	Nickel
Paba acid	Zinc	Cobalt
Biotin	Aluminum	
Folic acid		

and 16 amino acids

YOGURT

Yogurt has enjoyed a recent popularity as a low calorie food. That should not be the only thing to recommend this fine product of the Balkans. It has the consistency of custard and tastes like buttermilk (unless you buy the flavored brands—and watch what else is added besides flavoring!). Many people find it necessary to cultivate a taste for yogurt. The same can be said for beer, whisky and alcohol! So get busy. It helps the intestinal tract and acts as a natural antibiotic.

At bedtime yogurt helps promote sleep due to its calcium content. It is also used as an external beauty treatment. If applied to the face and left on overnight, the protein, calcium, and acid content is beneficial to the skin.

Yogurt contains all the same nutritional elements as milk.

LECITHIN

Lecithin is not well-known to doctors; they need to be introduced to it. Aside from the virtues we mentioned earlier, it helps prevent heart attacks by keeping cholesterol in a liquid state. We don't ordinarily eat many foods with lecithin and our blood runs short of it while cholesterol collects on the walls of arteries. There they can harden and cause the arteries to become inflexible, like steel pipe. The blood pressure rises and the pathway eventually becomes totally blocked.

The most common source is in soybeans.

You will find lecithin in egg yolk and soybeans. You can buy lecithin granules, which are made from soybeans. In the egg yolk, lecithin and cholesterol occur together. Inside the body lecithin dissolves the cholesterol and prevents it from piling up in the arteries.

Vitamins are also helpful in controlling your cholesterol level. This includes particularly vitamins B12, E and C.

LOW BLOOD SUGAR

Blood sugar—also called glucose—has been compared to fuel because it gives you energy and vitality. When your body converts starches to sugar, some of it is burned immediately for energy and the rest is stored in the liver and in muscle tissue to be used between meals. In this manner the glucose level of the blood is maintained at a proper level throughout the day.

An inadequate supply of blood sugar can lead to emotional disturbances by impairing the proper functioning of the brain. When the blood sugar content is low, all tissues *except* the brain can draw on fats and proteins for energy. The brain has no stored fats available and thus is dependent upon blood sugar for food and oxygen.

So don't go overboard and cut out all fats from your diet; your body needs *some*. Too little is just as bad as too much. Instead, do things like trimming the visible fat from meat before eating. Substitute unsaturated fats for the saturated ones. Use cold-pressed vegetable oils (from Health Stores) for cooking, instead of solid fats. Use vitamins B, C and E in your diet because they are helpful in preventing high cholesterol. Also try to maintain a serene disposition because stress interferes with the chemistry of the body. A great deal of the valuable food you take in can be lost to your system by the mere intervention of stress and anxiety, because it will be passed right on through and be evacuated as waste material without ever being used.

A suggested diet for people with low blood sugar would concentrate on the following:

- All meats, fish and shellfish.
- Eggs, milk, butter and cheese.
- Nuts (except between meals).
- Natural peanut butter (non-homogenized).
- Weak tea.
- Soybeans and soybean products.
- Natural bread (starch-free).

LIVER

Women who eat liver find it nourishes their skin and hair from the inside. It has more nutritional value than any other single food and is a rich source of vitamins, minerals and protein to supply energy and fight fatigue.

Liver contains:

Calcium.
Phosphorus.
Iron.
Nicotinic acid.
Vitamin C.
Vitamin B1.
Vitamin B2.
Vitamin B12.
Vitamin A.

So there you have six wonder foods. With just these six foods you could revolutionize your body's appearance and its functioning. The potential is almost staggering in its possibilities. **Stop and** consider for a moment: by applying this knowledge of nutrition and utilizing these foods, you can largely control the way you feel and the way you look the rest of your life!

Is it too much trouble? What's the alternative?

RECOMMENDED FURTHER READING:

"Secrets of Health and Beauty," Linda Clark, 1970, Devin-Adair Company.

"Stay Young Longer," Linda Clark, 1968, Devin-Adair Company.

"Let's Get Well," Adelle Davis, 1965, Harcourt, Brace & World, Inc.

"Feel Like a Million," Catharyn Elwood, 1965, Devin-Adair Company.

"Foods For Glamour," Jack La Lanne, 1961, Prentice-Hall, Inc.

"Eat, Drink and Be Healthy," Agnes Toms, 1968, Devin-Adair Company.

"Encyclopedia of Natural Health," Max Warmbrand, M.D., Groton Press, 1962.

CHAPTER FIVE

THE NATURAL WAY TO HEALTHY HAIR

WHAT DOES HAIR NEED TO LOOK ALIVE?

Beautiful hair is healthy hair; it's as simple as that. Or it should be. Beauticians make their living concealing the lack of health in many people's hair. Let them become wealthy from other people; become your *own* beautician. Within yourself lies the power to give yourself healthy, radiant hair; hair that's soft and shiny and bouncing with vitality; hair that women will envy and men won't be able to forget.

All that's necessary is knowledge and determination. You must learn what hair *is,* what it needs to live, and what will harm it. Armed with that knowledge, you will then see what the benefits are of giving your hair what it really needs, and the perils of denying it the proper nourishment. It shouldn't be hard to muster up the determination from then on!

Hair is a year-round crop which you grow in the soil of your scalp. The first thing you must remember is that the scalp is *skin.* It is not some unusual variation of what you usually refer to as "skin." It may be concealed by hair, but it is the same material, requiring the same kind of care and kindness as the rest of your skin.

The "soil" called your scalp is watered and fertilized by the same bloodstream that feeds the rest of your skin. What's wrong for any other part of your body is wrong for your scalp also.

Your hair is made of protein, as is the rest of you. That fact is only mentioned here so that you can dispel any misconceptions you may have acquired that different rules will govern the care of the scalp's skin than those governing other parts of the body. A lack of iron and copper, for instance, causes a pale and unhealthy bloodstream, and hair cells—like others—will go begging for nourishment.

A strand of hair is composed of a series of cells, and its color is derived from a pigment present in some of those cells. Each one of the perhaps 100,000 individual hairs on the average person grows out of a tiny pocket in the scalp called a follicle, at the bottom of which is the papilla, or root from which it grows.

It is through this papilla that the blood supply comes for the hair's nourishment. Each follicle has one or more oil glands opening into it under the scalp's surface. It is the oil from these glands which preserves the hair and gives it its gloss.

In a healthy person, hairs reach "old age" every two years and they fall out. They are automatically replaced by new ones. If you are *not* healthy, this replacement will not take place and you will have hair loss and eventually baldness. Additional factors which influence the rate of hair loss are excessive dandruff, tension, uncleanliness, metabolic disorders and certain hereditary factors.

A word about *tension*. Tension makes normal hair go dull and limp. It makes dry hair dryer and oily hair even oilier. As we keep saying throughout this book, learn to relax. A tense or anxious person is doing damage to his hair as well as other parts of the body. Try taking a 15-minute catnap at least a couple of times a day. You might place two small pads of cotton which have been soaked in cold water or witch hazel and place them over your eyes and relax. Be sure your feet are slightly elevated.

Winston Churchill was in his late sixties and fighting a three front war in 1942, but he still found time to take a short nap during the afternoon. Are you really busier than he was?

You might alternatively try sitting upright, placing both elbows on a table or desk and gently but firmly cupping your palms over your eyes. Stare into the blackness of your hands and try to think of nothing for a minute. Let all the tension and worry flow out through your eyes into your hands and elbows and down onto the table. Or use the slant board mentioned earlier.

People are accustomed to judging the health of a dog or cat or horse by its coat; whether it's shiny or dull; whether or not it seems to have life. Yet they give no thought to the possibility that their own hair could be just as much a sign of their own health or lack of it.

They realize that if the animal has a dull coating of hair, something must be wrong with its diet. Why don't they make the same connection with their own hair and diet? It probably has something to do with Man's Vanity: we like to think we are more complicated organisms than mere dogs and horses.

But our face is not separated from our body—it's a reflection of it. So too with our hair. It's all part of a unified and sensitive organism.

There are three principal causes for dull hair and dry, scaly skin:
Lack of vitamin A.
Lack of unsaturated fatty acids (fish and vegetable oils).
An underactive thyroid gland.

Cod Liver Oil is capable of curing all three situations. It has vitamins A and D, unsaturated acids and is also rich in iodine—for balancing thyroid activity. A daily dose should improve your skin and hair within a month or less. Your hair should have a new sheen and your skin a new and pleasing glow.

As a matter of fact all fish are rich in iodine, and iodine is very important to good circulation. And good circulation means plenty of nourishment for the scalp.

Iron is also vital to the growth and health of the hair. Here is a handy list of some of the best sources of iron:

Chicken.	Oysters.
Lean smoked ham.	Graham bread.
Roast leg of mutton.	String beans.
Lean roasted veal.	Green peas.
Loin of pork.	Spinach.
Molasses.	Broccoli.
Asparagus.	

And don't neglect the vitamin B-complex. Try including wheat germ, whole wheat bread, rice, yogurt, liver and eggs in your daily diet, if you aren't already.

HOW NOT TO TREAT HAIR

Hair problems can be caused by what you *don't* eat as well as by what you do. By the same token hair can be helped by avoiding certain foods as well as by eating certain ones. To have good hair, you should avoid carbohydrates, processed foods, soft drinks, coffee and cigarettes.

If you have oily hair you should also avoid chocolate, nuts, butter and fried foods because they all increase the production of sebaceous oils. If you have dry hair you must exercise caution in selecting your permanent wave lotions, your bleaches and any detergent shampoo.

You must beware of continual teasing of the hair, and overuse of hair spray and even the wearing of tight hats. All have a role in slowing down your circulation, discouraging new hair growth and in causing your hair to fall out. It is not the best policy either to wear your rollers around for long periods or to bed at night.

Continued washing with soap or commercial shampoos can result in the loss of calcium, phosphorus, iron, and nitrogen from your hair. If you feel you must use a commercial shampoo, at least choose one that does the least damage to your hair.

HOW CAN YOU SAVE YOUR HAIR?

No one should rely completely on her hairdresser for complete care of her hair. It's *your* hair and it's attached to *your* body. The problem has to begin with you and so does the solution. Only you can feed your hair the necessary *daily* ingredients of nutritious diet, fresh air and exercise.

Here are four steps you can begin taking immediately to put your hair on the road to recovery:

1. Watch your diet. Choose nutritious foods. Anything that will build up the proteins in the rest of the body will also benefit the hair.

2. Be sure your scalp is sufficiently acid. Skin which itches is alkaline. That itch is your body's way of reporting to you that it is lacking in acid. Apple cider vinegar and water will do the trick.

3. Always use a shampoo which tests as acid on Nitrazine paper.

4. When reconditioning hair, particularly dry hair, use an ordinary mayonnaise. The helpful ingredients include egg (for protein), vinegar (for acid), and vegetable oil. Apply the mayonnaise after you have shampooed and dried your hair. Then shampoo lightly again and rinse with apple cider vinegar.

A famous Nutritionist, Jheri Redding, offers this formula for conditioning dry scalp and brittle hair:

½ oz. apple cider vinegar.

½ oz. glycerine.

3 oz. polypeptides (available at some health stores and beauty salons).

½ oz. corn oil or wheat germ oil.

Shampoo the hair with an acid-balanced protein shampoo. After the second soaping, towel dry and apply the formula above, leaving it on the hair for at least 20 minutes to penetrate the hair shafts. Then rinse and set.

Well-known beautician Frances Schoenecker recommends a home wave set to help give body to your hair. You can find flax-seed in your health store and using a cup of it (ground or whole) add it to three cups of water. Bring to a boil. At this point you can dilute with water to the desired consistency.

Egg white may also be used, but you may not like the "heaviness" it leaves the hair with. A set lasts longer with brush rollers, but you may have a problem with fuzziness from the brush ones. If so, use smooth, plastic rollers.

You will also add body via either a protein wave-set or a protein hair spray.

Redding also suggests skim milk as a wave set, but you must not rinse it out, but rather allow it to dry. If this isn't enough body for you or doesn't last long enough, make a paste of dried skim milk powder with water and apply it to your hair as a pack. Leave it on for 20 minutes.

The basic essentials to remember about hair reconditioning are as follows:

1. Brushing and massage every day with a natural-bristle brush. Healthy hair stands out from the head rather than lying plastered against your scalp.

2. Shampoo once a week (or every two weeks) using natural herbal shampoos. If not available, use castile with a lemon or vinegar water rinse.

3. Never use anything except natural permanents, tints and hair aids.

4. Use proper nutrition and supplements.

Brushing

Brushing is a million dollar secret of hair beauty. Your grandmother wasn't so far off when she did the ritual 100 strokes a night. Brushing not only stimulates circulation, it also helps normalize both dry and oily hair.

Dry hair benefits because brushing stimulates the oil glands and distributes oil from the scalp to the ends of the hair, while oily hair gets the excess oil distributed more evenly throughout the hair.

When selecting a brush, be sure to select one with animal bristles because they're soft. You should never use a stiff nylon brush due to its harshness.

Every day brush your hair thoroughly in order to cleanse the scalp between shampoos and remove the skin which is normally "shed." This daily ritual also spreads any excess scalp oil evenly, relieving dryness. The circulation also helps nourish the hair. When brushing, always lower your head toward the floor and use an outward wrist motion.

When brushing oily hair, cover the bristles with clean gauze or cheesecloth to absorb the oil. In the case of dry hair, wrap an old nylon stocking around your brush bristles. This will catch the dandruff.

Cleaning the brush involves placing it with bristles down in lukewarm water (hot water will soften the bristles) mixed with ammonia. Then rinse in clear, cold water. And don't forget to dry the bristles in a warm, dry place with the bristles down.

For a stimulating scalp massage, hold your fingertips firmly against the sides of your head and move the scalp itself with your fingers. Slowly knead your scalp, going over the entire head that way.

A scalp massage is a must before you shampoo. Try this for five minutes: Use your fingertips in a circular motion, placing both hands on your scalp, palms flat up against it, with your fingertips about an inch apart. Now push your hands together so that the fold of the scalp is pushed up between the fingertips. Repeat over every part of the head until the whole scalp feels loosened.

Another effective exercise is pulling the hair to bring more blood to the roots and thicken the scalp tissue. Start at the front of your head and pull, lifting and pulling with interlocked fingers.

Combing

Combs irritate the scalp and should be used sparingly. When selecting one, be sure it's sturdy, yet flexible; one with rounded teeth that won't scratch your scalp. When you are combing, always hold a handful of hair at a time and work out from the center to the ends. Back-comb as little as possible and remember to change the part in your hair from time to time.

When cleaning a comb, soak it for 15 minutes in a solution of hot water with a few tablespoons of ammonia. Scrub the comb with a nailbrush until it's all clean. Then rinse with cold water and set aside to dry.

SPECIAL PROBLEM AREAS

Dry Hair

Covered oil glands produce a lack of scalp oil and cause dry hair. One of many recommended means of combatting this is to use a natural pore-cleaning agent, along with a heat cap. This will achieve a dilating and perspiring effect.

You could also wash with a mild, oil-based shampoo and warm water. Follow this up with a cream rinse to restore oil and give hair its highlights and manageability.

Alternatively, rub castor oil into the scalp at bedtime and shampoo in the morning. At first, do this twice a week and then taper off to every two weeks. Some women may not wish to leave the oil in all night. In that case, rub the oil into the scalp thoroughly before you shampoo and then steam it in by pressing hot towels on the head.

Some women like to massage warm olive oil into the scalp, steam it with hot towels and then shampoo.

Since the prime purpose of everything that you do for your hair should be to keep it lubricated, an occasional hot oil treatment is a very effective preshampoo conditioner.

The best hot oil treatment starts with placing warm olive oil (or castor oil) in a cup. Using cotton pads, apply the warm oil to your scalp. Then wrap your head in a hot towel. Continue these hot towel treatments for at least twenty minutes before massaging the oil into the scalp and hair. Wrap your head in a fresh hot towel and keep it on for at least an hour. Then shampoo at least three times to remove all the oil.

Oily Hair

Women with oily hair should shampoo a minimum of twice weekly in warm water using a soap-based preparation to whip up a sudsy lather. Give yourself three sudsings and then rinse with warm water. Next, open a can of beer and let it go flat. Pour the beer over your hair, massaging it gently into the hairs. Rinse again in clear water and set.

Another possibility is to mix ½ pint of ethyl alcohol, ½ pint of warm water and 30 grains of quinine and rub it into the scalp every other night.

Good results can also be obtained by adding a spoonful of ammonia and a little borax to two quarts of warm water and using this for an after-shampoo rinse.

An alternative to such frequent shampooing is to clean the hair every other week by shaking cornmeal into it and brushing it out. A kitchen salt shaker is the best means. And don't forget to spread newspapers on the floor to catch the meal as it's brushed out!

Dandruff

Dandruff is a normal skin function. Matured cells and food waste products are sloughed off by the body as what we call dandruff. It is only excessive dandruff that is a problem. The regular shampooing will cleanse away the normal amount of dandruff.

It is not advisable to use a dandruff-remover shampoo because they are so powerful in disinfectant and antiseptic action that their prolonged use will lead to the removal of hair too. A good shampoo should be sufficiently antiseptic to control dandruff except for the unusual cases of infected follicles and pores.

Try mixing equal parts of vinegar and water, parting the hair and applying the liquid to the scalp with cotton pads. This also cleans and stimulates the scalp. This can either be done separately or as a before-shampoo cleaning.

Another anti-dandruff trick is to beat one raw egg lightly with a fork and then rub it thoroughly into the scalp instead of a shampoo. Rinse out with warm water and repeat once a week.

For really unbeatable, entrenched dandruff, try placing in a bottle one ounce of sesquicarbonate of ammonia, ½ pint of spirits of rosemary and one and a half pints of rose water, shake thoroughly and apply to the scalp with absorbent cotton pads, as you part the rair. Then brush the hair.

If you're interested, among Vermont countryfolk one tablespoon of corn oil taken morning and evening with meals is used successfully to control dandruff.

Baldness

There are three million bald women in the United States today and over four million more are well on their way. These are the generally-agreed-upon reasons for bald women:

- Too vigorous brushing with harsh brushes.

- To much sun.

- Infections and other diseases.

- Lack of scalp exercise.

- Emotional tensions.

- Allergies to certain hair preparations (dyes, sprays).

- Drugs.

- Too much shampooing with alkaline soaps (losing protective acid mantle).

- Detergent shampoos which strip the oil glands under the scalp.

- Dandruff-removing shampoos which remove hair also.

- Harsh chemicals in permanents, bleaches, tints and rinses.

- Poor nutrition.

Baldness is, in many cases, reversible. Here are a few treatments that have proven successful in renewing hair growth. Bear in mind that anything that makes hair healthy will also contribute to its growth.

One treatment is to rub coconut oil on the scalp every day. Another is to take several tablespoons of honey and thin it out by adding brandy and stirring them together. Massage into the scalp and leave for several hours. Then shampoo out.

You might also stew a pound of rosemary in a quart of water for 5 to 6 hours, then strain and add one half-pint of bay rum. Rub this into the roots of the hair night and morning.

Or you might rub kerosene on the head and leave it overnight and shampoo thoroughly in the morning. It leaves no odor.

Blondes should put lemon juice in the rinsing water after a shampoo, or else wash their hair in stale beer. Brunettes would be advised to add vinegar to the rinsing water.

Falling Hair

Researchers have determined that a man's hairline recedes about an inch at age 30 and, with proper care, tends to remain there. In woman the same thing doesn't happen until age 50.

Thinning spots on the scalp can be caused by suffocation of the scalp, which has various causes.

Sometimes certain rinses leave a residue, coating the scalp with a very plastic-like film. This seals off activity of the scalp almost completely. If you don't shampoo more often than every two weeks and you don't use a vigorous scrubbing action, a state of impaction builds up causing the scalp to become hard and sore, and choking off the hair roots. If circulation to the roots is completely cut off, the roots will die and a bald spot will be created.

Inositol is the key to this situation. When animals are put on a diet lacking inositol, their hair falls out. If the vitamin is added again to the diet, their hair grows in again in a few weeks. It has also been known to return hair growth to bald men. Black strap molasses and sunflower seeds are the best sources of inositol.

If your hair is falling out in patches, it is best to see a dermatologist as it might be a thyroid malfunction.

Jheri Redding claims that the following treatment stops cases of falling hair in over 85 percent of the situations. Mix 4 oz. of red cayenne pepper with a pint of 100 proof vodka and shake several times. Strain it— preferably through a nylon stocking—until the liquid is free of pepper. Apply the mixture to the threatened scalp areas each morning and evening for two weeks. Within six weeks there should be new hair.

There is a famous folk remedy for falling hair which is nothing more than alternating applications of castor oil and white iodine over a period of four days. On the first and third days the iodine is applied to the scalp directly with a swab of cotton as you part the hairs. In between do the same with the castor oil. Use just enough to penetrate the scalp, as otherwise you will get a sticky mess.

On the fourth day, massage a little more of the oil into the scalp and then steam your head by wringing out a very hot towel and wrapping it around the head. Repeat the hot towel about four times, then shampoo.

Other folk remedies consist in doing things like rubbing the juice of a lemon into the scalp, or mixing a combination of a teaspoon of salt, a pint of brandy, and one and a half grams of quinine and rubbing that on the scalp each night.

Gray Hair

The causes of gray hair are not always the same for each person. We don't yet know all the reasons, but among the ones that have been established, there are:

- Stress.

- Poor circulation to the scalp.

- Anemia.

- Lack of iodine or copper.

- Lack of B vitamins.

- Lack of unsaturated fatty acids.

- Mal-nourished glands.

Several nutritional researchers have found that copper in the diet is an important element for reversing gray hair in humans.

Black strap molasses is unusually rich in copper. Amazing results have been reported from people taking a mixture of black strap molasses, natural honey and apple cider vinegar.

If you are already taking vitamin B, remember that it is water-soluble and therefore a large intake of water may be washing the B right out of your system before it has had time to do its work.

KEEPING YOUR HAIR LIVELY AND HEALTHY

While most hair problems are correctable, prevention is still the best method to follow. Proper diet must go hand in hand with daily hair care.

Many hairdressers try to interest their customers in various food treatments, using food directly on the hairs. For instance, lemon juice helps cut down on oiliness, can be used as a mild bleach or to bring out the highlights in hair. Eggs give body and sheen to hair when used in a shampoo. Vinegar will help make the hair soft and easy to manage, especially after a tint. Olive oil conditions the scalp and hair. And don't forget camomile tea; it's one of the oldest known applications to bring out natural highlights.

People have also been rubbing beef marrow into their scalps for centuries. There are many more exotic-sounding things like fox grease, skunk oil, goose grease and bear's grease which, whatever your feelings toward them, are of proven efficacy over the centuries.

Just as important as beginning to use natural foods and products on your hair may be, don't forget to analyze the other things you have been doing for and to your hair over the years. Become a label-reader.

For instance, *hair sprays*. Some are cheap, some are expensive, but very few are bargains in the long run. Most of them contain varnish, shellac, or a lacquer emulsified in water. Sometimes a little perfume is added; sometimes a little lanolin.

The lacquer-based sprays will immediately seal up the pores. This has the effect of sealing-in the sebaceous and waste materials, causing both hair roots and the pores to become impacted, interfering with the normal skin functions and can stunt hair growth. Itching, scaling and cysts will result.

Don't compromise the health of your hair for the convenience of the hair sprays. If you really feel you can't get along without them, there are safe ones on sale at health stores, and from beauty salons which carry natural beauty products.

Many *hair dyes* are quite harmful and border on the poisonous. They can enter the body via the hair shaft and play havoc with your general appearance and your health. Tint poisoning is another name for aniline-derivative poisoning which can lead to baldness in some people. Aniline is a colorless, poisonous, oily liquid used in making dyes.

Many people are allergic to aniline, which is cumulative in the system. Yet most hair colors contain aniline. The exceptions are "metallic salt" colors, henna and the pure vegetable hair colors (which contain no harmful ingredients at all).

It is preferable to make use of herbal hair colorings; here are a few examples.

To *darken* the hair: Use left-over tea leaves. Place one tablespoon of dried sage leaves and four tablespoons of tea leaves in a sauce pan. Add enough water to make one pint and simmer for half an hour. Strain and then throw away the leaves. An alternative to tea leaves is rosemary. Massage gently into the scalp and gray hair once or twice a week.

For *blonde* hair: Add three or four tablespoons of dried camomile flowers to a pint of water. Boil 20 minutes and then strain when cooled. Be sure to shampoo first before using to be certain the head is free from oil. Then use this mixture as a rinse by pouring it over your head while you bend over the sink. Repeat several times.

If you are trying to avoid getting a "mousy" shade to your blonde hair, boil a quarter of an ounce of camomile flowers and a quarter ounce of quassia chips about ten to fifteen minutes in just enough water to make a reasonable amount of rinse. Use it once or twice a week.

Bleaching is another problem entirely. Chemical bleaches will burn out difficult-to-replace protein cells, indicated by a dryness and lack of elasticity. The hair can become hollow and lose its sheen. This is all a senseless waste. Natural bleaches can be made from vegetable materials such as tomatoes and alfalfa, which contain no harsh acids, chemicals or peroxides. Yet they are every bit as effective.

Not all *permanents* are safe, either. Thioglycolic acid is a chemical substance used in permanents and has been known to lead to thioglycolic poisoning. This results in hair loss, cramps, lymph disorders and scalp itch.

A few words about *shampoos* and shampoo procedures. Always remember to brush before shampooing. This will free your hair of any tangles.

In order to shampoo properly, you should lather with a non-chemical shampoo two or three times. Allow the last lathering to soak a few minutes in order for it to "lift" the dead skin cells from your scalp. Then you should rinse thoroughly.

Remember that detergent shampoos are harmful to the life of both the hair and the skin because they strip the scalp's oil glands of precious lubricating oils. You will find many fine herbal shampoos available at your local health store, but if you aren't satisfied with them or if there *isn't* such a store convenient to you, a good vegetable oil shampoo will serve equally well—and safely!

If at all possible, avoid shampooing in hard or chlorinated water. Rain water is ideal, but most of us have to settle for store-bought pure spring water.

And don't shampoo under the shower. Sure, it's faster, but the force of all that water pounding down on your scalp isn't good for your hair. Especially when it's chlorinated and probably fluoridated too!

As a matter of fact, some women in Europe never shampoo at all. Instead they rub oatmeal into their scalps and comb it vigorously throughout their hair to remove the dirt and oil. What does their hair look like? Well, they are so beautiful in the hair department that they are the ones who sell their hair for manufacture of the wigs the American women feel they must wear. That should say enough right there. If not, the women of India "wash" their hair with clean potter's clay or soapnut powder.

Did you ever try an egg shampoo? Scandinavians have been taking them for generations and finding it a sensational beauty aid for any kind of hair. It's such a *natural* way to help your hair.

Separate two or three eggs into the yolk in one dish and the white in another. Whip the whites to a peak. Mix the yolks with a tablespoon of water until the mixture is creamy. Now mix the whites and yolks together in an egg froth. Wet your hair with warm water and towel off the excess moisture. Apply the egg froth to your scalp with your fingertips and massage gently until the egg is thoroughly worked into the damp hair. Be sure to rinse with cool water. Repeat the process until you have used all the froth. Then rinse until every bit of the egg is gone from your hair. Pat it dry.

There are also various natural *rinses* you may wish to try.

Blonde: Strain the juice of two lemons through cheesecloth. Mix with an equal amount of lukewarm water. Without rinsing let the hair dry in the sun. For dry hair, rinse with cool, clear water.

Redhead: Take a mild shampoo followed with a tea rinse (to enhance the highlights and to give long hair an extra bounce). Brew some camomile tea as per directions on the package. Strain this through cheesecloth and mix with a pint of water, then pour it through your hair and rinse with clear water.

Brunettes: Mix 4 tablespoons of cider vinegar with 3 glasses of water. Massage the mixture gently through your hair and follow with clear, cool water to remove the vinegar odor.

When *drying* your hair don't massage it with a rough towel. Rather squeeze the water out gently and fluff dry with the towel.

Better still, if possible, dry in fresh air. Squeeze the excess in a Turkish towel and then step outdoors and swing your hair dry. You can combine this with a torso-swinging exercise to kill two birds with one stone.

You might also combine this with a short sunbath, which is not only safe, but a beauty tonic as well.

You shouldn't shampoo more than once a week. If there is an itching in between shampoos, clean the scalp with witch hazel on small cotton pads.

For a *general hair tone up* any of the following suggestions would be in keeping with natural beauty arrived at through natural means.

Create your own shampoo by taking a bar of pure castile soap and shaving it finely with a knife. Add water to the shavings and heat over a low fire until the soap is melted. Let the amount of water be determined by how thick you want the mix.

There is a trend among some hairdressers in New York to use lemon juice, milk, eggs, vinegar, olive oil, tea and stale beer.

RECOMMENDED FURTHER READING:

"Secrets of Health and Beauty," Linda Clark, 1970, Devin-Adair Company.

"Stay Young Longer," Linda Clark, 1968, Devin-Adair Company.

"Feel Like a Million," Catharyn Elwood, 1965, Devin-Adair Company.

"Beauty and Health the Scandinavian Way," Gunilla Knutson, 1969, Avon Books.

"Natural Beauty Secrets," Deborah Rutledge, 1966, Avon Books.

"The Natural Way to Beauty and Health," Carlson Wade, 1968, Bantam Books.

CHAPTER SIX

A NATURAL-LOOKING SKIN—ORGANICALLY

1. *The Composition of Your Skin*

WHAT IS SKIN MADE OF?

Your skin is the largest *organ* of your body. It is not just some nice-looking material spread over your insides to keep them from falling out! Nor is it some sort of celestial cosmetic sprayed onto your skeleton to make you look better. It is an integral part of you and has many useful functions besides helping your looks.

It is an organ which performs certain jobs and in return it is "fed" by the body, via the circulation of the blood. As a matter of fact, the skin receives about a third of all the blood circulating through your body.

The average adult body contains 17 square feet of skin which weighs about six pounds. That's more weight than either the brain or the liver. A piece of skin the size of a quarter contains a yard of blood vessels, 4 yards of nerves, 25 nerve ends, 100 sweat glands, and more than three million cells.

WHAT ARE SOME OF THE SKIN'S FUNCTIONS?

The skin protects the body against bacterial invasion and against injury to sensitive tissues within the body. It protects the body from harsh sunrays and loss of moisture. It also serves as an organ of perception for the entire nervous system, reporting such sensations as pain, pressure, and heat and cold. It helps to regulate body heat and to lubricate the hair.

WHAT IS THE SURFACE COMPOSED OF?

The skin's surface has millions of tiny pores and hairs, covering almost all the body, excreting oils from the skin glands to keep the surface lubricated. This outer layer, called the epidermis, is constantly being shed as an inner layer replaces dead cells with new ones. A complete renewal of the cells in your body takes place every 7 years.

WHERE ARE THE NERVE AND SWEAT GLANDS?

In the second layer of skin, called the dermis, lies the nerves, sweat glands, blood vessels, nerve receptors, hair follicles, and oil glands. There are literally millions of these sweat and oil glands busy keeping the skin soft and flexible. They are most numerous on the chin, forehead and nose, but they exist all over the body.

Also in this layer of skin are 150 million "papillae" containing the nerve fibers and special nerve endings (such as the fingertips and lips) which give us a sense of touch and the "feel" of things.

WHAT IS IN THE THIRD LAYER OF SKIN?

The subcutaneous (third) layer of skin is made up of fat globules and blood vessels and serves to give a smooth and springy base for the skin. The third layer lies next to the bones and muscles.

DOES THE SKIN ACTUALLY BREATHE?

In the sense that air and nourishment are taken in through the skin and waste material is excreted through it, yes. As proof, witness the several reports of people who painted themselves from head to toe with gold or silver paint for costume parties and became ill and died because their skin was unable to breathe.

Tests on rats (and more recently on people) have indicated that vitamins can be absorbed through the surface of the skin. If further tests bear this out, it could have revolutionary possibilities for the cosmetic industry. Rats were fed a diet lacking in vitamins B and D and soon developed symptoms of a lack of those vitamins (see Chapter Two for a list). Then these vitamins were applied to their skin daily, and in such a way that they were prevented from ingesting the vitamins by licking themselves. In a short time they lost the symptoms and recovered robust health. They could only have received those vitamins from the skin's absorbing them.

2. Nourishing Your Skin

IS IT POSSIBLE THEN TO "FEED" YOUR SKIN?

It's not only possible, you *must* do it! Remember, the skin is an organ. Your heart, liver, eyes, etc. are all organs and you know what you must do to feed them and what happens if you don't. Skin must be fed too; primarily from the inside, but also from outside of it. No skin can reach its potential beauty, nor retain it for long without proper nutrition internally.

SPECIFICALLY WHAT VITAMINS DOES THE SKIN NEED?

The skin requires vitamins A, B, C, and E, as well as the mineral silicon and large amounts of water.

WHY IS VITAMIN A NECESSARY TO THE SKIN?

Without vitamin A, the skin gets dry and scaly, the scalp forms abscesses, dries out and loses hair. At least one type of skin eruption is due to this deficiency. A shortage of "A" can cause enlarged pores, blemishes and rough dry skin. If you have problems with rough skin and blackheads, you will benefit from increasing your intake of vitamin A. It can be added to your diet by yellow or green vegetables and fruits, as well as in supplementary pills.

WHAT HAPPENS WHEN YOUR SKIN LACKS VITAMIN B-COMPLEX?

If you are deficient in any of the B vitamins, you increase your chances of eczema or dermatitis. Vitamin B is noted for making strong, relaxed nerves which help circulation. Low circulation will lead to dry, lifeless and sallow skin. Lack of "B" causes redness, tenderness and ulcerating of the skin at the corners of the mouth.

B vitamins have also contributed to curbing excessive oiliness on the skin, and are important in dealing with the dark blotches which appear on people's skin after age 40 or 50. These deficiency signs will usually disappear after a while when a tablespoon of brewer's yeast is taken with every meal.

WHAT ARE THE SIGNS OF VITAMIN E DEFICIENCY?

Tired-looking skin is the most obvious sign of a lack of vitamin

E. The skin looks so tired because it lacks oxygen, and E stimulates circulation which brings oxygen to the tissues.

WHY IS VITAMIN C NECESSARY FOR THE SKIN?

If vitamin C is missing from the diet, there is damage to the structure of connective tissues. Vitamin C is noted for strengthening the tissues underlying the skin and making them firmer. Vitamin C also prevents easy bruising caused by the destruction of capillaries under the skin.

WHAT IS SILICON?

Silicon has often been called the "beauty mineral" because it is essential for keeping skin from getting flabby, and for the growth of rich hair and natural sheen. It also promotes growth and strengthens nails. It is found in apples, honey and avocados.

WHY IS WATER ESSENTIAL TO THE SKIN?

Nutritionists have called water the "non-vitamin vitamin." Your body is composed of 70 percent water. Since it helps to create energy, it is considered to be a valuable food. It lessens anxiety about pressing problems because it relieves brain congestion.

Water helps your body free itself of toxins generated through emotional upheaval. It dissolves hardened "debris" in your tissues and bloodstream by picking up discarded particles and carrying them away. It helps to stimulate sluggish circulation.

You should drink 8 glasses of cool, crystal water a day—preferably spring water—to flush poisonous substances out of your system. Some nutritionists suggest a glass every hour.

HOW BAD IS SUGAR FOR THE SKIN?

Refined white sugar is particularly destructive to your skin beauty by causing blemishes, falsely satisfying the appetite, and filling you with valueless foods, and thereby denying your body the enriching food it needs. The blemishes and pimples are products of the bacteria which thrive in an undernourished skin and which are fed by the sugar.

3. *Basic Skin Types*

WHAT HELP IS THERE FOR DRY SKIN?

Before applying make-up, use a bland soap to clean your face, and rinse with warm water. Avoid hot water at all times as it contributes to your drying condition. And don't give in to the temptation to scrub too vigorously since the dry skin is usually fine-textured and can't take too much friction. Rinse your face with cold water and pat dry with a towel, using a gentle blotting action.

You should try to steam your complexion once a week because, since your pores stay tightly closed, your skin fails to perspire freely. Open them with steam and close them after with cold water.

Every ten days to two weeks apply the juice of a honeydew melon onto the skin as you would a cold cream. Just mix the juice with regular white petroleum jelly. Some women prefer to rub the face with castor oil or olive oil.

Your dry skin is probably also aggravated by steam heat in the wintertime. It would therefore be best to sleep with the windows open an inch or two. It is also well to leave them open during the day to get fresh air for your lungs and skin.

HOW CAN SKIN-MOISTURE LOSS BE PREVENTED?

There are a number of steps you can take to prevent this. Avoid excessive sun-tanning or exposure to strong winds. Avoid strong chemicals which tend to dry out the skin. Avoid drying soaps. Skin is naturally acid, while most soaps are alkaline and drying (detergent soaps are even more drying and irritating).

Avoid overheated rooms as the moisture has been removed from the air by the heating.

Include unsaturated fatty acids in your diet, since they tend to stimulate the production of natural oils from inside the body. Adding cod liver oil and lecithin to the regular diet is most helpful.

WHAT CAN BE DONE FOR OILY SKIN PROBLEMS?

Oily skin is aggravated by a diet too rich in fats, sweets, and spices. Emotional upsets can contribute, too; as can overly-long exposure to hot water. Try using a medicated soap about three times a week, working up a rich lather with hot water. Use a fairly rough washcloth to increase the circulation produced. Be sure to let the lather dry before scrubbing. Work over the oiliest areas, around your forehead, chin and nose.

Rinse with cold water and then wind up with a brisk astringent to close the pores. You should remove excess oil which builds up during the day by carrying in your purse some astringent pads.

Give yourself a facial steam even as often as three times a week to unclog those pores and avoid blackheads and unsightly blemishes.

Another treatment is to bathe the face with *wine* once every two weeks in the morning and the evening. Use white wine for fair skin, red for olive complexion.

Some women bathe their face once every ten days or two weeks with the juice of fresh strawberries or fresh cucumbers The juice could also be mixed with petroleum jelly and applied as a skin cream (see "Dry Skin" above).

Over-oily skin has also been found to yield to vitamin B6, which can be found in brewer's yeast. You can buy brewer's yeast in powdered or tablet form.

To make an effective cleansing cream for oily skin, mix 2 ounces of white paraffin (soft), ¼ ounce of stearic acid, 1½ ounces of white wax, 1 dram of borax and ½ ounce of distilled water. Apply nightly to the skin in a liberal fashion, let stand for 30 minutes, and then tissue off.

If you would prefer a cleansing lotion, try mixing 2½ oz. of glycerine, an ounce of camphor, 4 ounces of spiritus odoratus and 2 ounces of distilled water. Apply it with cotton and wipe off.

A suggested astringent which you could mix at home contains one dram of borax, 2 ounces of glycerine, 2 ounces of alcohol, 1½ ounces of rose water, and two drams of a tincture of benzoin. Mix it together and apply with cotton after washing, and let dry on the skin.

WHAT IF THE SKIN IS BOTH OILY AND DRY?

Some people have skin which is dry near the sides of the face but oily in the center. The first thing they must do is wash the oily sections more often than the dry. You'll need a man's old-fashioned shaving brush in order to work up a rich soapy lather. Put the lather on the oily patches with the brush and allow to dry. Then rinse it off with *hot* water and finish it off with cold—*ice* cold. Pat dry with a clean towel and apply an astringent to the oily parts.

The dry skin areas should be lubricated with a moisturizing cream or lotion by day and a complexion oil at night. Follow all the rules for dry skin, for those patches. Remember to eat a diet balanced for both conditions.

4. *General Rules for Skin Care*

IS IT POSSIBLE TO WASH TOO MUCH?

No. Your skin takes a lot of punishment from all the auto pollution and the soot and grime in our urban air from factories and incinerators, etc. Your pores get impacted with dirt and this leads to blemishes and wrinkles. Anything you can do to counteract these forces of destruction, by all means employ them! The best way to keep your skin clean is with regular washing, so don't worry that you could wash too much.

WHAT IS A DAIRY WASH?

Women have been bathing in warm milk for centuries. With milk prices what they are today, you will probably have to make do with just washing your face in it. Mix the same amount of melted butter as room-temperature milk and use it as a cleansing lotion. Wipe off with tissues. It's another way of "feeding the skin" from the outside.

IS A WINE WASH SAFE?

Of course; wine is made from grapes, not chemicals. Just before retiring, wash your face with some wine, splashing it on and letting it soak. Then tissue it off. Dark wine for dark skins, light wine for light.

ANY SPECIAL HINTS FOR THE BATH?

Try to make your daily bath a pleasant ritual; one that you look forward to, rather than something else that must be squeezed into the day's activities. Oily skin will require a fluffy bubble bath, while a bath oil will be helpful to the dry skin.

If you found the milk wash enjoyable or stimulating, you may decide to hang the cost and have a milk *bath*. Actually it needn't be as expensive as dumping several gallons of fresh store-bought milk into the tub. There are readymake milkbath powders at drug and department stores, and there's always powdered skim milk.

Milk baths create a very feminine feeling of sheer luxury and help to smooth all types of skin.

As for the daily ritual, naturally you start by running warm water into the tub and then adding your bath oil. Have your moisturizing cream or lotion on a nearby chair or stool. When the water is ready, take your time as you step in and lie down. Relax completely; luxuriate as you apply your beauty aid. What a perfect way to begin or end a day.

If you are *starting* your day with this bath, it is important that you take the phone off the hook while you bathe. Nothing can shatter this luxurious mood quicker than the incessant jangle of an impatient telephone!

You may wish to try an oatmeal bath for a change. Pour about a pound of fine oatmeal or oatmeal flour into a tub of warm water. The oatmeal has certain oils which soothe and lubricate dry skin. Bran is an alternative to oatmeal. After either bath it's still advisable to shower in order to remove all traces of the bran or oats.

French women use a bath bag similar to our tea bags. They make a bag out of cheesecloth (about a yard of it) and fill it with bran or oatmeal or almond meal and let it soak in the bath water the way tea bags soak in the tea water. Alternatively, they would use the same idea for a washcloth, only in this case they would include all three meals:

  1 lb. fine oatmeal.
  ½ qt. clean bran.
  2/5 lb. powdered orris root.
  ¼ lb. powdered castile soap.

Another fine old recipe for toning up the skin and refreshing the body is an herb vinegar bath. You can make one by taking a dram or two each of rosemary, rue, lavender and camphor and soaking them in a pint of white wine vinegar for several hours. Strain off the herbs and add the liquid to the bath water.

Those are just a few of the more exotic, yet natural, organic additions you can make to your daily bath for health and variety. Now let's go back to the ordinary, everyday type of bath.

After you have dried off, cool your entire body with generous splashes of your favorite cologne. Then rub all the hard-to-clean spots (elbows, knees and heels) with a paste made of cleansing grains mixed with water. Scrub hard enough to remove dry, flaky skin.

If you usually shave your legs at this point in your ritual, you can remain in the tub if you use a safety razor. Just remember to shave upward and follow with a smooth coat of cold cream. When you use an electric razor, try a preshave lotion to reduce razor pull.

WHAT IS A SAUNA?

A Sauna is a thermal bath which produces a high, dry heat. Saunas have been used in Finland for a thousand years. They are so popular there that estimates indicate there is one Sauna for every six Finns.

The temperature gets up to 200 degrees in the wood-walled rooms but the humidity never gets to be more than 10 percent because it is such a dry heat. It causes you to perspire freely and opens the pores, stepping up circulation. And it bakes a pleasing warmth into the very marrow of your bones. Are they beneficial? The greatest advertisement for them is the Finnish women! Their complexions are legendary the world over.

ARE COMMERCIAL LOTIONS AND CREAMS ACCEPTABLE?

Remember that emollient creams can only act on the surface of your skin; they cannot go deep enough to absorb adequate moisture from the body and they do not strengthen facial muscles.

WHICH NATURAL ONES ARE VALUABLE?

To stimulate sluggish skin you should dissolve an ounce of boric acid in 2 ounces of witch hazel and wash your face with it several times a day. It will help return that look of youth to your skin.

English Royal women have partaken of "barley water" for centuries and helped them preserve their tradition of beautiful women in the court.

The recipe for barley water goes like this: Place a half cup of pearl barley into 2½ quarts of boiling water and simmer at a low heat, with the lid on, for one hour. While this is on, squeeze two lemons and six oranges, keeping the juice. Strain the cooked barley water into a bowl and add brown sugar or honey and the rinds from the lemons and oranges. Allow to stand until cooled. Remove the rinds and add the juice and store in the refrigerator. Drink with a meal.

Many women find it hard to choose between the benefits of cucumber cream and cucumber juice. The cream is made by mixing 6 ounces of cucumber juice, 3 ounces of rosewater and 6 ounces of witch hazel and making it into a paste. Rub it into your skin the way you would any cream.

The cucumber juice itself is prepared as follows: Wash and cut up cucumbers and put in an earthenware or porcelain dish. Pour boiling water over them until they are covered. Place the dish over a low fire and simmer 30 to 40 minutes, being careful not to scorch them. Strain off through a collander.

WHAT'S SO DANGEROUS ABOUT COSMETICS?

Manufacturers have learned that women are virtual pushovers for any product which promises to improve their appearance. The profit margin is fantastic because they seldom cost very much to make and can be sold for high prices in staggering quantities. A profit of 2,000 percent is reportedly not unusual.

As with other aspects of our civilization, the manufacturers—in their haste to make money—have often ignored the safety factor when it comes to the ingredients.

For instance, ammonium sulphide—which is used in deodorants—has been known to cause some peovle to itch, swell, and break out in a rash and their skin to crack.

Indelible dyes in lipstick causes cracking, drying and peeling on some women's lips. Preservatives in some cosmetics give an allergic reaction at times. PVP, which is contained in some hair sprays, has been found to cause lung disturbances.

For your guidance in choosing cosmetics, here is a list of toxic chemicals which have been found in commercial cosmetics:

Aluminum salts
Ammoniated mercury
Barium salts
Beta-naphthol
Boric acid
Cresylic compounds
Formaldehyde
Lauryl alcohol sulphates
Mercuric bichloride
Phenolformaldehyde resins
Phthalates
Phenyllenediamine compounds
Polyethylene glycols
Propylene glycol
Salicylic acid
Sulphur
Thioglycolate
Zinc salts

That list was provided in 1963—nine years ago—by Dr. Irwin I. Lubowe in his book *New Hope For Your Skin.** It was not represented as a complete list at that time, and—knowing the industry, and judging by the chemical "advances" in the food and drug industry since then—it is probably only a fraction of what such a list would include today.

IS THERE A SAFE POLICY?

Three good rules to follow when buying cosmetics would be to use an absolute minimum of commercial cosmetics, use only a reputable manufacturer's goods, and when you find a preparation you like and can use safely, stay with it.

Better yet, try to develop a natural glow from the *inside* through proper nutrition, plenty of exercise, fresh air and rest, and use a minimum of makeup.

*Irwin I. Lubowe, *New Hope For Your Hair,* 1963, E. P. Dutton & Company.

HOW DO YOU TEST COSMETICS FOR ACIDITY?

You can purchase Nitrazine paper in any drug store. This will be yellow when you buy it. Immerse it into the cosmetic you are questioning (unfortunately you can only do this after you have bought it!) and watch the color of the paper. If it remains yellow, the preparation is acid and safe to use on your skin. If the paper turns gray, blue or purple, it indicates alkalinity of some degree which may prove harmful.

Use this test for checking alkalinity in lotions, creams, shampoos, wave sets and soaps.

WHAT ARE SOME HOMEMADE COSMETICS?

When you buy a commercial preparation containing a petroleum such as minerals oils, this cannot possibly be absorbed by the skin, so how could it "nourish" the skin? It can't. It can only make it *look* better, or *feel* better. Whereas on the other hand, edible fats *can* result in the useful replenishment of skin oils, you should try using things like salad oils as a skin cream. Cold-pressed soy oil contains many elements which occur naturally in skin tissue.

Experiment with these home creams and lotions; find the one that works best for you.

Camphor Cold Cream

½ oz. spermaceti
½ oz. white wax
3¼ oz. oil of sweet almonds
¼ oz. camphor
1½ oz. distilled water
15 grains borax
4 drops oil of rose geranium

Mix spermaceti and wax together and add the almond oil. Stir and add the camphor. Dissolve the borax in distilled water and add the rest. Stir until it is well-mixed and beginning to thicken. Remove from the fire and stir until it begins to cool, and add the geranium oil. Continue to beat until cold.

Clover Cream

1 oz. spermaceti
1 oz. white wax
5 oz. sweet almond oil
1½ oz. rose water
20 grains powdered borax
5 drops essence of clover

Dissolve borax in rose water and add clover essence. Using a porcelain pot or double boiler, melt wax spermaceti and almond oil and then remove it from the heat. Add the rose water with the borax and clover in it, then beat until cold and firm.

Creme Marquise

¼ oz. white wax
2½ oz. spermaceti
1½ oz. oil of sweet almonds
1½ oz. rose water
1 drop of attar of roses

Shave the wax and spermaceti and melt, then add the almond oil and heat gently. Remove from the fire before it boils and add the rose water and perfume. Beat until creamy (but not hard).

Creme Simon

2 oz. cocoa butter
2 oz. lanolin
2 oz. glycerine (unless your skin is allergic)
2½ oz. rose water
1½ oz. elderflower water

This is good as a skin food.

Orange Flower Skin Food

½ oz. spermaceti
½ oz. white wax
2 oz. sweet almond oil
1 oz. lanolin
1 oz. coconut oil
3 drops tincture of benzoin
1 oz. orange flower water

Melt the fats over a low fire or in a double boiler. Then remove a double boiler. Remove from fire and add benzoin and flower water, beating with a beater until fluffy and cold.

Perfumed Cleansing Lotion

  4 oz. oil of sweet almonds
  1 oz. lanolin
  1 oz. white petroleum jelly
10 drops violet extract

Melt the fats over a low fire or in a double broiler. Then remove from the fire and beat until cool, adding the perfume drop by drop.

Strawberry Cream

  ½ oz. white wax
  ½ oz. spermaceti
2½ oz. sweet almond oil
 ¾ oz. strawberry juice
  3 drops benzoin

Wash and drain the fresh strawberries, mash them and strain the juice through muslin or cheesecloth. Heat the wax, spermaceti and almond oil in a double boiler. Remove from the fire and add the strawberry juice very quickly. Beat briskly until fluffy, then add the benzoin as the mixture begins to cool. Mix it in well then keep in icebox at least until it hardens. Apply every night.

Virginal Milk

  1 pint rose water
  ½ oz. simple tincture of myrrh
10 drops glycerine

Stir into the rose water, drop by drop, the benzoin, then the myrrh, and then the glycerine. This is recommended for cleansing the skin of all dirt and makeup.

With those few examples you can see how easy it is to make your own cosmetics. The best reason is that you can include only those ingredients which you have learned are best for you from your own experience.

5. Problems of Skin in General

WHAT CAUSES ACNE?

The precise cause is still unknown; it probably has to do with the mysterious hormonal changes occurring during adolescence. It is basically a malfunction of the sebaceous glands.

WHAT IS THE PREFERRED TREATMENT?

For serious acne or eczema, you should of course consult a dermatologist. Otherwise, washing gently once or twice a day, using a medicated soap and followed by an astringent, should keep it under control. In addition, here are some related remedies you can experiment with safely to find the one that is best for your skin.

Pimples

Mix equal parts of mutton tallow (which is pure lanolin), glycerine and castor oil. Melt on a mild flame to blend it smoothly, let it cool and then keep in a glass jar. Keep applying it to the pimples until healed. Of course this will not work very well if you continue eating large quantities of valueless foods and small quantities of nutritious ones.

Another way is to mix 36 grains of bicarbonate of soda, one dram of glycerine and one ounce of spermaceti, making a smooth paste. Rub onto pimples and leave on for fifteen minutes. Then wipe off with a soft cloth, leaving a slight film on the face.

Blackheads

A very old recipe for combatting blackheads is to mix a pound of powdered oatmeal, 8 ounces of powdered almond meal, 4 ounces of powdered orris root and an ounce of powdered castile soap. Each time you wish to use it, take about a tablespoonful and slightly moisten it with hot water to make a paste. Rub it gently into your blackheads with your fingertips and then rinse with cold water.

Red Blotches

Cod liver oil is best for this, used plain or as part of a commercial ointment (for baby's diaper rash). It works on all kinds of blotches and rashes.

Boric acid is also good. Dissolve it in boiling water and let cool before patting on. Calamine lotion is the old favorite: pat on and leave.

Large Pores

Buttermilk is useful because of its astringent effect. Pat it on your face with your hands or with absorbent cotton. Let it dry for ten minutes or so and then rinse off with cold water.

Another possibility is to mix equal parts of vinegar and hot water. When cool, you can use it as a facial wash with the cotton pads.

For centuries English women have used a few drops of spirits of camphor in cool rinsing water to tighten up pores.

Freckles

Try mixing 3 drams of lemon juice in 2 drams of borax and dissolving in an ounce of hot water. Pour in an ounce of red rose-petals and leave soaking for an hour. Strain through a cheesecloth and let stand for 24 hours. Then add an ounce of glycerine and pat onto your freckles.

PALE SKIN INDICATES WHAT?

Pale skin indicates the body is starving for acid. There is a new soap available which is high in protein, contains acid, but includes no "soap" at all. Yet it cleans and sudses wonderfully.

WHAT IS THE BEST TREATMENT FOR SUNBURN?

Take any commercial vinegar and pat it lavishly on the sunburned area. It takes the sting out and is very soothing.

Most people tend toward calamine lotion applied liberally and allowed to dry. You might also cut up a fresh cucumber into small pieces and let them soak for five or six hours in milk. Then pat it on the burn—if you can wait that long!

To get at the problem quicker, you could dissolve a pinch of baking soda in a cup of ordinary milk and start right in patting it on the sunburned areas. That is probably the "best," in the sense that you can work with it right away (and not have the smell of vinegar about you). They all work and all are natural ingredients.

CAN ANYTHING BE DONE FOR AGING SKIN?

Wrinkles are caused by a deficiency of vital food elements resulting in a devitalization of the skin. It is further aggravated by frowning and facial grimaces. What people usually think of as being "to be expected," is merely the result of incorrect diet and care of the skin.

New research indicates that a moist skin retains its pliability because it is the *water* in the skin which keeps it young-looking, not the lanolin, olive oil or petroleum applied to it. When the skin loses this moisture, it becomes hard and brittle, not when it loses its fat.

Aging skin not only gets drier and drier, but it also loses its plump succulent look. It begins with most people at around age 40. The skin's elasticity disappears; oil glands decline in number (except in nose and forehead); things start to happen which we resign ourselves to as "old age creeping up on us."

Prolonged exposure to sun and wind and chemicals may cause premature aging. The ocean-going fishermen, the Eskimos, and the tribesmen of the desert lands all show dried wrinkly skin early in their middle years. Living in an overheated house or apartment can cause similar skin-moisture loss.

IS IT EVER TOO LATE TO HELP AGING SKIN?

Skin is never too old or too young to improve. You can actually "roll back the years" by using natural skin-youthifying remedies. Here are a few of the best.

Exercises

The secret of restoring youthfulness to the skin is in friction. You can polish and rub out wrinkles by using your palms and your fingertips, using any of your preferred cleansing lotions to prevent chafing. Stretch the skin between the first and second fingers of one hand. Rub with the fingers or palm of the other— slowly at first.

Another technique is to do a facial exercise while wearing an egg mask (see below). Close and contract one eye as hard as you can. At the same time, lift and tense the entire face on the same side in the manner of a wink and a smile. Do this about 25 times a minute for each eye. Start with a few times a day and work up to a few dozen times a day.

Cream

Mix three ounces of lanolin, 10 drams of olive oil and 4 drams of castor oil. Apply it as a night cream.

Egg White Mask

Beat one egg to a light froth and apply to the wrinkled portion of your face with a shaving brush (or complexion brush). Allow it to dry and set for 5 minutes. Then rinse off with warm water. Repeat several times a day.

An egg white mask was supposed to be the secret of Cleopatra. Her variation was to include a tablespoon of honey and the whole thing was to remain on for 30 minutes instead of five. Take your pick.

WHAT ABOUT HORMONE CREAMS?

Most recent reports are encouraging. They indicate that estrogen-treated patches of skin have shown an increased water content, resulting in fewer wrinkles. Progesterone has been found to increase the number of oil glands in aging skin. The glands produce a film called sebum which protects the skin against abrupt changes in temperature or humidity, and helps to maintain the moisture content of the surface skin. There are creams containing both estrogen and progesterone.

Hormone creams should be approached with caution as there is some danger (when large doses are administered) that they can be absorbed through the skin.

Women who have yet to experience menopause do not derive much benefit from hormonal creams because they are still producing their own hormones. In women over 50 and under 80, it usually takes 10 days for results to show. Then after a month or two, there is no further benefit from them.

6. *Problems of Specific Body Areas*

WHAT IS THE BEST FACIAL MASK?

Either of the egg masks already described. While they remain on the face you can actually feel the impurities being drawn out of your skin, feel it tightening and the pores closing. Afterward, your skin feels baby-soft, and looks clean and fresh. Don't feel as if the yolks are wasted because you can use them in scrambled eggs or to make a richer egg salad.

The egg mask is the very oldest facial mask in the world; trust it! Use it!

IS THERE A RECOMMENDED FACIAL MASSAGE?

Swedes seem to have the best approach—and they have acquired a reputation for excelling in massages of all kinds.

1. Start at your collarbone (at the point where it joins the base of your neck) and run your fingers gently over your throat in a hand-over-hand motion.

2. With the backs of both hands under your chin, flutter the back of your fingers against your chin, working from the center outward and upward toward the earlobes.

3. Placing your index finger of one hand at the point where the corner of your mouth meets the line running down from your nostril, hold that skin slightly taut. With the fingers of the other hand, work the skin upward and outward in a circular fashion.

4. Starting at the sides of your nose with your index fingers, curve your hands up and out along the cheekbones all the way up to your hairline.

5. Using the pads of your fingers, stroke gently over the eye area. Work from the inside tip of the eye upward and outward toward the eyebone.

6. Use a circular motion on the forehead, nose and chin. This will stimulate, but not stretch, the skin.

7. Wind up by drumming all ten fingers lightly over your entire face, alternately patting and lifting.

ARE FACIAL SAUNAS SAFE?

Of course they are. You can buy an electrically powered facial sauna, but it is cheaper to make your own. All you have to do is fill a washbasin with boiling water and make a tent out of a terry-cloth towel draped over your head as you bend over the washbasin. Steam your face that way for at least 5 minutes.

If your skin is oily, you may want to lather your face first with an antiseptic soap and let it dry before steaming. When you come out, splash cold water on and pat dry. Then apply an astringent.

For those with dry or normal skin, you could apply a rich cream or complexion oil to your face and throat before you start. At the end, splash cold water on and dry with a patting action.

WHAT IS THE BEST TREATMENT FOR THE HANDS?

It's harder to hide any problems that may develop on the hands, because you so seldom can hide them. You don't wear makeup or stockings so whatever you have will show. And wouldn't you know—that's the first place to start showing signs of age. Part of the reason is that household chores are hardest on delicate hands; too many bleaches, detergents and scouring powders.

The only way to counteract the results of washing is by rubbing creams and oils on them. One kind of oil you can make yourself is to mix equal parts of glycerine and rose water. If your skin is allergic to glycerine, pure lanolin will do.

An old-fashioned recipe for keeping hands soft and white involves boiling a teacupful of oatmeal in a gallon of water for an hour, straining it and then bathing the hands night and morning in it.

For really problem hands, you might try the "Oatmeal Glove." Buy a pair of oversize cotton gloves, rub oatmeal into your hands each night and wear the gloves to bed.

WHICH WAY TO BEAUTIFUL FEET?

The most important, but perhaps the least able to be followed, advice is to wear shoes that fit and do not give you corns and calluses. We seem to be getting away from the fashion of stiletto high heels which used to tilt the foot at an unnatural angle and throw the whole body off balance. But pointed toe shoes and flat shoes are still much in evidence and doing their damage.

The first thing you should do is to throw out all shoes that fit improperly. You can't have beautiful feet that are covered with corns and calluses.

If you have corns already, go to a podiatrist to have them removed and then don't wear the shoes that caused them.

Calluses are another story. You can keep them under control by rubbing them with pumice stone every time you bathe. Afterward massage them with oil, glycerine, lanolin or any good cream. Rubbing the whole foot once a week with warm olive oil is a recommended beauty treatment. You should massage the oil into the skin around the nails and the callused areas.

WHAT SHOULD BE DONE FOR SHOULDERS AND ARMS?

An old English custom was to melt 2 ounces of yellow wax together with 4 ounces of honey and 6 of rose water in a double boiler. Blend them together by stirring. Remove them from the fire and immediately add an ounce of myrrh. When it cools, rub it thickly on the skin and leave on all night (or all afternoon if you're going to an evening party).

HOW CAN SPLIT NAILS BEST BE COMBATTED?

The growth rate of fingernails is reportedly accelerated by adding protein and vitamin A to the diet, so that's one clue as to what can be done. Eating gelatin has always been known to be good for strengthening. You can buy it in a store and make your own "Jello" out of it.

The most common cause of soft nails—which is more prevalent in women than men—is contact with harsh chemicals. Women are more regularly handling laundry detergents and dish-washer detergents, bleaches and ammonia, as well as putting chemical cosmetics on their hands. In most cases of the cleaning chemicals you could wear rubber gloves. It still would do no harm to soak your nails in olive oil once a week.

COULD YOU RECOMMEND ANYTHING FOR CARE OF THE EYES?

The most important thing for eye care is to get sufficient sleep each night, as the eyes will reflect lack of sleep sooner than any other part of the body. In Spain and Switzerland, women still squeeze a drop of orange juice into each eye each morning to keep them clear and bright. Beyond that, here are several recommended eyewashes you can make yourself:

1. Make a weak tea and dip two gauze pads into it. Then lie down for 10-15 minutes, with the pads on each eye. This will rest the eyes and brighten them and is not harmful.

As a variation, steep green tea in rosewater for the same effect. Or some women prefer witch hazel.

2. Make a camphor eyewash by dropping a small amount of spirits of camphor into tepid water. It's soothing and refreshing for tired eyes.

3. Mix a little boric acid in boiling water and allow it to cool. Then use it with an eyecup when your eyes are inflamed or tired, or for dust specks that may be caught in them.

4. A very old recipe for eyewash consists in mixing a teaspoon of boric acid with 15 drops of camphor in two thirds of a cup of water, boiling hot.

RECOMMENDED FURTHER READING:

"Secrets of Health and Beauty," Linda Clark, 1969, Devin-Adair Company.

"Stay Young Longer," Linda Clark, 1968, Devin-Adair Company.

"Feel Like a Million," Catharyn Elwood, 1965, Devin-Adair Company.

"Beauty and Health the Scandinavian Way," Gunilla Knutson, 1969, Avon Books.

"Natural Beauty Secrets," Deborah Rutledge, 1966, Avon Books.

"ABC's of Skin Care," Dodi Schultz, 1969, Bantam Books.

"The Natural Way to Beauty and Health," Carlson Wade, 1968, Bantam Books.

CHAPTER SEVEN

WHO SAYS YOU *HAVE* TO GROW OLD?

There is a myth popular in our culture to the effect that when a person passes forty, particularly a women, she is no longer "young" and should "act her age." The woman who is past forty is made to understand that she is "over the hill" as far as various things are concerned: attractiveness to men, youthful fashions and amusements, and the possibility of appearing young.

It is "understood" in our culture that your hair will gray, wrinkles will appear, skin will sag and dry up, eyes will fail, hair will thin and a thousand indefinable aches and pains will develop and have to be borne with the good grace of "a middle aged person."

Doctors will listen to your complaints and nod sympathetically and then admonish you to "cut down" on something or other which you are used to doing. He'll mumble something about you not being as young as you used to be and prescribe some pills or drugs which, if pressed, he will have to admit aren't going to do more than give temporary relief because, in his words, "Your body has begun its decline into old age, and more and more of these things are going to occur until some vital part gives way and your body stops altogether."

If he has heard anything in his medical "education" about the importance of good nutrition and plenty of exercise he will betray a precious lack of appreciation for it, because he will give you certain prohibitions which will effectively reduce the meager amount of exercise you may now be getting and he will prescribe a diet and a medicine that will further complicate your damaged digestive system—necessitating further returns to him.

When you get this kind of "return business" from a TV repairman or a garage mechanic (after they fix one thing something else goes) you usually get suspicious and change repairmen. But how often do we question the doctor's expertise? Perhaps not as often as we should.

A really expert mechanic (and how few there are!) and one who might be taking an altruistic interest in the condition of cars in general, or at least a very active interest in the ones belonging to his regular customers, would not simply ask you "What's wrong?" and then go fix it. Nor would he just give it back to you with an admonition not to drive through potholes so fast or not to let the battery run down. He would want to know all about your driving habits, what kind of starts and stops you make, what routes you regularly use that may be in bad repair, where you garage it and what kind of fuels and oils you feed it.

Only a mechanic with *that* kind of an interest in your car could really get at the things that might *soon* go wrong with it and thus save you much heartache later on. Only he could persuade you to change your driving habits to insure a longer life for your car. Only he could really help you keep it looking "young" and sounding "young." Otherwise you are doomed to an endless succession of repair bills throughout the life of your car, unless you are a trained expert who not only knows how to shift and steer, but also knows proper handling and preventive maintenance for the car.

Most doctors, unfortunately, seem to be like the average mechanic when it comes to taking care of the body. They wait until you have a problem, ask you "What hurts?" and then focus their expertise on that area to the exclusion of others. They prescribe a remedy for that ailment and usually inquire no further into your living habits, eating habits or related aches and pains that aren't yet of sufficient magnitude to justify a visit to the doctor.

When was the last time *you* were asked by a doctor to list the foods you eat regularly so that he could determine if you were getting too much of something or not enough? The answer lies partly in the time involved. The ratio of sick people to doctors to doctors' hours in this country is very bad. The other part of the answer is that doctors are primarily educated in how to repair broken people, not in how to keep them whole.

In a survey of almost 300 medical schools which give nutrition courses to medical students, the *longest* course in Nutrition (well above average) was only a total of 5 hours! That's five hours out of the 4,000 odd hours those students spend in learning to be doctors. How could anyone learn enough in that short time about the fantastically complex organism known as the body and how it utilizes nutrients?

No wonder that doctors are not prone to put sufficient weight into the area of proper nutrition for keeping a person well or making him well after an illness. It was never impressed upon them in medical school, and after that they are so busy with their day-to-day work that it's not possible to keep up with all the latest experiments being done all over the world. They probably tend to keep up only with things in their own specialty within medicine. General practitioners probably do not subscribe to the same magazines and trade journals or professional magazines as nutritionists and thus are also kept in the dark on nutritional developments. We pay a high price for this professional exclusiveness.

But, doctors to the contrary, your hair needn't turn gray or remain gray; wrinkles need not come so soon in life; your skin need never lose its vitality; your eyesight need not abandon you; nor need you bear the thousand and one indefinable aches and pains. No one can guarantee you will live forever, but you *can* retain your beauty and your staying power far beyond what people generally think should be the time of senility and feebleness.

What makes women feel that 40 is such a highwater mark anyway? Why should women older than that feel like "has-beens?" As a matter of fact, Wallis Simpson was forty years old at the time the King of England resigned his throne for her, "the woman I love." Many of the most romantic women in history have been over forty. So you needn't *feel* like a has-been, and neither should you allow yourself to *look* like one.

Perhaps the reason French and European women of 40 are still considered very much "in the running" in romantic sweepstakes is that they retain their interest in sexual matters longer than their American counterparts. Or rather, they are not afraid to express or to indicate an interest, whereas in America we still have, due to our Puritan heritage, a residue of popular feeling that sex is for "young" people; that a "mature" married woman should be more concerned with her family and her home than in retaining the interest of or an interest in the opposite sex.

One consequence of this is that American women seem to exert more effort into keeping up the appearance of their home than in themselves. They let their appearance slip because they assume if they are 40 they should look it or else people will talk, and feel she is "abnormal," or "sex mad." This is nonsense. Taking care to retain your youth need not imply anything of the sort.

WHAT ARE THE CAUSES OF AGING?

Learning the causes of the aging process in our bodies should help to clarify why it is possible *not* to age; at least not obviously nor precipitously.

Biochemists have determined that what we call "aging" is merely improper nutrition carried to such an extent, and over such a period of time, as to lead to the damage of tissues and organs, or their starvation. In other words, we are continuing to make withdrawals from the bank account of our body without making sufficient deposits to cover them. Since the "bank" has known us a long time and since we are its only customer, it is reluctant to close us out and turn us over to the authorities (the undertaker). It keeps sending us "dunning notices" indicating the amounts that we owe (pains, aches and diseases) but we seem to misunderstand. As soon as we pay up one bill, we go right back to writing bad checks again. Finally there is a day of reckoning.

It starts in the blood, usually. When the supply of nutrients in the blood begins to drop (due to inadequate intake of the right foods), the body borrows the necessary nutrients from the supply on hand, stored in the tissues.

When the reserves which had been stored up in the body's tissues become exhausted, the body will begin to "raid" the reserves in vital organs. These reserves in the tissues and organs have been set aside by nature on the premise they will only be used when special strength or endurance is required, not to maintain the day-to-day functioning; that's supposed to be done by the daily diet.

Try to imagine the military preparedness pipeline. It stretches from the steel mills to the factories to army bases to warehouses to the front line. Prior to a war, the army will "stockpile" various materials, clothing and equipment over and above what wears out and must be replaced each month. As long as those factories keep pouring supplies into the pipeline, the army can use what it needs and store the excess.

When a war breaks out, the army rushes to meet the attackers and uses up supplies at a faster rate, so the factories have to produce faster to meet the demand.

Now suppose the enemy throws a blockade around the country so we can't get the raw materials the factories need. Or say the workers at the factory go on strike so that nothing is being produced. For a while the army can get by on what it has in the forward camps. Then it has to dig into the warehouses; first one and then another.

One by one the warehouses all over the country are emptied, but still the army uses up equipment and ammunition every day. One day one of the regiments will send out a supply truck and it will come back empty, even though it visited warehouses for other regiments. What will happen? That regiment will have to surrender to the attacker.

A good general may be able to stop up the breach in the line by shifting other regiments from elsewhere on the line to the point of the breakthrough, but that regiment too will be understaffed, underfed, and underequipped. It won't be able to hold the new line very long. Pretty soon the enemy will overwhelm the army.

We would consider those striking mill workers to be very callous individuals indeed for not heeding the appeals from the army for more materials; for not giving up their selfish interest and working for the common good in this emergency. And we would be right in so doing.

Well, *you* are those striking factory workers if you are not giving your body (the army) the materials it needs (vitamins, minerals, proteins) despite the calls for help (aches and pains).

If that army were somehow successful and won the war by the skin of its teeth, the first thing it would do would be to rebuild and re-equip its regiments; then it would stockpile against the next onslaught. And you must do the same. You must maintain a high rate of production to not only keep up with your day to day requirements, but also stockpile against those extra demands.

Unfortunately when those warehouses close to the front line are raided for supplies, no one will realize right away the seriousness of the predicament. So too, when your body first begins to "rob Peter to pay Paul," the few symptoms that show up will probably not be recognized as a nutritional problem. Yet your resistance to infection is dropping, your ability to bear up in adversity will decline, and—more important for a book emphasizing beauty—subtle and undesirable changes will begin to take place in your personality: wrinkles, frowns, impatience, lack of skin tone and vitality.

It is said that diabetes has begun five years before the patient recognizes anything wrong. Old people are susceptible to broken bones, not because they are "old" but because the calcium deficiency has finally reached a critical stage where it couldn't take the punishment. The bones broke because the person ate a calcium deficient diet for a critical number of years, not because he was getting old.

There is even a theory that old people do not break arms or hip bones because they fall, but rather that they fall because a bone snaps first. Either way, the mineral deficiency has finally taken its toll; the bank is finally refusing to honor a check; the naked army is surrendering on one front.

Most people expect their bodies to degenerate automatically as they get older and to develop things like arthritis, heart attacks and cataracts. But "age" doesn't cause those things; they are created by a persistent strain put on an organ that is weakened due to lack of nutrition. We die when one vital part which has been deteriorating gives up or wears out sooner than the others.

"Old Age Diseases" require decades to develop and are difficult to diagnose in a young person. Rather than be surprised at this statement, we should be surprised that with the nutritional punishment we give the body day in and day out, year in and year out, that it lasts as long as it does!

Remember: it is possible to be "old" at any age; all it takes is improper care of the body and lack of nourishment. Look at the victims of Auschwitz and Dachau. Those pictures should forever haunt us of very young people made to look very old by the simple device of mal-nourishing them (in every sense of the word) and taking away hope and optimism.

These symptoms, seen anywhere on the sidewalks of the U.S.A., are the S.O.S. signals of poor nourishment which, if unheeded, can develop into "old age" diseases:

Body

Overweight and flabby.
Underweight, undersize, or emaciated.
Flabby, drooping muscles.
Awkward coordination.
Poor posture (round shouldered and stooping or
potbellied).
Difficulty in walking.

Face

Drawn and worried.
Overanimated.
Hard and bitter.

Hair

Gray or fading.
Dandruff.
Falling hair.
Dry and brittle.
Coarse and hard to manage.

Skin

Permanent goose pimples.
Premature wrinkling.
Cracks in corners of the mouth.
Loose and pale.
Waxy and sallow.
Rough and dry.

Lips

Thin and tightly stretched.

Eyes

Bloodshot.
Granulated eyelids.
Dull, tired, or burning.
Crusting, or redness among lashes.
Watering or flinching at bright light.
Dark circles underneath.

Digestion

Poor, finicky appetite.
Constipation.
Gas.
Nervous indigestion.
Gastric ulcers.

General Observations

Sore joints.
Fatigues easily.
Irritable, moody, hard to get along with.
Poor memory.
Poor healing of wounds.
Sensitivity to cold weather.   .
Leg cramps at night.
Overly active.
Confusion.
Insomnia.
Trembling hands.
Headaches.
Lethargic.
Lack of attentiveness; attention wanders.
Restlessness.
Low resistance to infection.
Unnecessary worrying about improbable things.
Superficial hemorrhages, bleeding gums or nose.
Poor endurance.
Querulous.
Dizziness-prone.

None of these are natural conditions; none are inevitable. All are signs of some sort of nutritional deficiency which if not corrected will lead to the consequences we have been discussing.

TECHNIQUES FOR STAYING YOUNG

You cannot look good if you don't feel good. Whatever you are feeling is mirrored in your face; happiness, sadness, bewilderment, antagonism, vindictiveness or contentment; it's all there.

The same goes for constipation and headaches, as well as for a general happiness at being alive today.

It has been observed that most people only feel well about half of the time. The rest of the time they have some sort of ache or complaint whether persistent or occasional; major or minor. It's still there and it keeps them from being and looking healthy.

If you want to retain your youth (and why shouldn't you?) you must retain your health, and in our society this takes no small effort. Time has to be set aside for exercise; time is spent locating and frequenting the nearest health store; time must be spent planning meals intelligently instead of just heating up what happens to be around; time must be spent on beauty care, etc.

The American Medical Association's Committee on Aging has come up with a formula for living longer and better. It is well worth remembering:

- A balanced diet of more protein, vitamins and fluids; fewer fats and calories.

- Regular elimination of waste products.

- Adequate rest of both mind and body.

- Pursuit of interesting and specific recreational activities.

- A sense of humor.

- Avoidance of excessive emotional tension which leads to personal ineffectiveness.

- Mutual loyalty of family and friends.

- Pride in a job.

- Participation in community affairs.

- Continued expansion of knowledge, wisdom, and experience.

It went so far as to summarize this list by reducing it to *two* rules: the preservation of energy and a high degree of motivation. Under the first heading would come both exercise and nutrition, which we have discussed at considerable length in this book.

One further word on nutrition might serve to emphasize its overriding importance. A nutritional doctor in Birmingham, Alabama, was called upon to treat 893 people who had been chronically ill and unable to work for years. He found they had no serious diseases, just vague complaints about digestive, nervous and mental ailments. The one thing they all had in common was a vitamin deficiency.

The doctor placed them all on a nutritional program which eventually resulted in the return to work of all 893 people! This doesn't mean that there are no such things as diseases, nor does it mean that certain foods will cure certain illnesses all the time. It only indicates that nutrition is a key element in maintaining and restoring health to "aging" people.

You might wish to try a Scandinavian beauty secret called the Beauty Cocktail. But you must make it a *daily* drink:

> 2 tablespoons of brewer's yeast
> 3 tablespoons of wheat germ
> ¾ glass of skim milk
> ¼ glass of fresh fruit juice

Mix it all in a blender and drink daily.

Equally important as proper nutrition is physical exercise. We stressed that combination elsewhere in this book for health and beauty, and we stress it again for retarding the aging process. Anything that keeps your body healthy also tends to keep it young, so get all the exercise you can; exercise every day.

Before you get out of bed in the morning, stretch the muscles and tissues of your body; contract and relax them; do facial exercises. Then take a cold shower and give your face a good massage. Finally, sit down to a good nourishing breakfast: apples, oranges, grapefruit, peaches, pears, plums or prunes—not some bland, valueless dry cereal, harmful pastry or valueless coffee. Give yourself a good start in the morning and you will approach the day in a much younger, anticipatory frame of mind which will brighten your face, and, particularly, your eyes.

If you have a bicycle, use it; if you don't, get one. There are few things better for firming and trimming legs, hips, buttocks and waistline than the exercise you get pedalling a bike. It's a great tune-up for your system and helps dispel nervous tension. Better still, it's a good helpmate to vitamin E for preventing heart attacks.

It's never too late to start cycling; people in Europe have been cycling to work far into their eighties and nineties. And it would certainly help the air pollution problem if more Americans cycled to work instead of driving their cars!

Skipping rope is another easy way to help your body stay young. Do 50 counts by an open door the first thing after rising each morning. It helps your breath control, your posture, legs, upper arms and torso. And it's fun! Remember all the hours you skip-roped as a little girl?

Having a positive frame of mind is also conducive to keeping young, so forget the past and look to the future. Forget your petty little grudges you may be holding against someone. What does it all amount to anyway? Don't drag along all the inconsequential hurts of the past. Live and let live. Yesterday is gone and can never come back. Today is already here and leaving fast. If you have things to do, get busy and do them. If you don't, *find* something that interests you and do it.

The AMA Committee on Aging suggested things like pursuing interesting and specific recreations, pride in a job, participating in community affairs, and continued expansion of knowledge and experience.

Nobody dies from work that they enjoy. And remember that worry kills more people than work ever did. Worry leads to fear, anxiety, hate, envy and jealousy, and it all shows in your face and in the tenseness of your muscles.

Learn to smile; see good in everything. If you have a pleasant expression, one of good cheer and good will, you will attract people favorably. It's pretty hard to smile without thinking pleasant thoughts. A smile is always good for relief of tension throughout the body.

Retain a healthy curiosity about people and places and events. Keep your own judgment and values, but be interested in learning what others are doing and thinking and why. Mixing with younger people and sharing their fun and hopes can be a fruitful way of keeping abreast of things. The "Generation Gap" we hear so much about is nothing more than the dividing line between those who think of themselves as old and those who know you are as old as you feel!

Lastly, get plenty of sleep and sunshine. Lack of adequate sleep leaves you tired and worn out in appearance. The sunlight has a wonderful purifying effect when you let its chemical rays bathe your face. Don't forget, that's your prime source of vitamin D.

DEALING WITH SPECIFIC AGING PROBLEMS

Wrinkles

People make their own wrinkles. Negative thoughts, repression of feelings, and pessimistic attitudes all tend to leave their marks on the face in the form of wrinkles.

You doubt that there is a direct connection between your thoughts and your facial tissues? What happens when you blush? A change of thought—the introduction of an embarrassing idea—has altered your heart's action in controlling the circulation to the face.

In addition, therefore, to smiling a lot more and thinking pleasant and positive thoughts, you ought to try rubbing the face daily with castor oil or olive oil (recommended by Cleopatra). You might try a facial sauna first. You could do the rubbing while soaking in a hot tub, as the steam from the tub encourages the oil (possibly cod liver oil, in this instance) to sink into the skin.

Some of the remedies mentioned in the chapter on skin care are also good for wrinkle-prevention, especially the honey and egg mask.

The best advice for wrinkle prevention is really a prohibition: avoid too much sunbathing. When it fades, a woman over thirty-five can look quite withered from her suntan.

Crow's Feet and Wrinkled Eyelids

Make a cream for crow's feet out of a pound of raw lanolin and a small bottle of sweet almond. Melt the lanolin in a double boiler, slowly adding enough almond oil to make a spreadable cream. It should be the consistency of rich cold cream.

Another technique, this one used by French women (does that make it sound more romantically authentic?) is to stretch the wrinkles away with your fingers and place adhesive tape over the spot where they were. Do this every night after you have removed your makeup, and sleep with the tape on.

Lines Under The Eyes

Holding your head perfectly still, look straight up and then straight down (only your eyes move). Look to the extreme left and then the extreme right. Slowly make a circle with your eyes: up, to the side, and down, to the side, and up. Repeat three times. Gradually increase to ten times.

You can also practice pushing your lower eyelids up toward your eyes with a very light pressure from your fingertips. Keep your face free of tension while you do this and be careful not to wrinkle your forehead. Lift both lids as high as you can slowly, then relax and try again.

The Chin Line

Imagine there is an apple hanging on a string from the ceiling and your hands are tied behind your back. Throw your head back and try to bite into it, using your lower lip to bite and your upper to hold the "apple" steady. You can feel the pull in the chin and neck muscles as you try about 15 times to bite that apple.

Gray Hair

A highly recommended home remedy for restoring hair to a close approximation of its original color is canute water, which can be purchased at drugstores.

Chapter Five of this book has additional information regarding gray hair.

Menopause

The better your daily nutrition, the easier you will get through this difficult time. Menopause involves many of the same symptoms as pre-menstrual tension and responds to the same treatment. For instance, since every gland and nerve is under a readjustment strain during menopause and is jangling like a combination of the doorbell and telephone ringing at the same time, B-Complex vitamins can act as a soothing influence on them to bring you some peace and quiet.

Here is a quick check list for the nutrients you need particularly during your menopause:

Vitamin A	For minimizing tension and irritability.
Vitamin B-Complex	For normalizing blood sugar and destroying excess hormones.
Vitamin C	For helping the body lose water safely.
Vitamin E	For helping circulation.
Calcium	For soothing nerves.
Lecithin	For feeding sex glands and helping the liver destroy excess hormones. It is a natural tranquilizer.

If you have a craving for something sweet, instead of eating sugary things eat protein or fruit. Sugar gives the blood sugar a boost temporarily, but then drops it lower than ever. Much of pre-menstrual irritability is due to low blood sugar.

HANDLING THE PROBLEM OF ARTHRITIS

As we have repeated throughout this book, good health is normal and disease is abnormal. It needs to be said over and over, because when a person looks around at our society he might think the direct opposite is true; that someone who dies at a ripe old age and had few if any illnesses was a person who somehow "put one over" on nature.

But all of nature is built on order, and man's body is no exception. If we take care to observe the rules of living, we enjoy good health. But if we ignore those rules or flout them, then disease—the body's protest against abuse—will result.

There are over 8 million arthritics in the United States. Indeed, it has been estimated that 97 percent of all Americans over 40 have some degree of arthritis.

What is it? It's an inflammation of the joints, usually accompanied by swelling. It can strike at any age, but it is most common in people in their 40's and 50's.

Many cases of arthritis are caused by infections, tumors and nervous conditions, but the principal cause seems to be a prevalent condition called "autointoxication." Very simply it means self-poisoning by means of not promptly eliminating poisonous waste products. In a word, constipation is the leading cause of arthritis.

When the bowels are not systematically and regularly evacuated, and the diet contains the sort of toxins contained in our typical American diet, the body slowly but surely begins to poison itself. The quality of the blood is diluted and the albuminous fluid in the blood which lubricates the body's joints becomes weaker and weaker. A lack of exercise further adds to the situation by reduction in the blood's circulation.

Nine out of ten adults are troubled by some degree of constipation after age 40. It has been identified as a leading cause in both rheumatism and arthritis.

In a normally functioning body, the waste expelled from the bowel is moist and thus carries in solution such things as sulphuric acid, phenol, skatol, indol, bacterial wastes and other poisons.

When constipation occurs, much of that poison-laden moisture is reabsorbed into the blood and lymph (the fluid that actually nourishes the body's cells). Thus these poisons are distributed throughout the body, resulting in pimples, headaches, eczema, colds, bronchitis, rheumatism and arthritis.

Waste matter must be expelled from your colon at least once a day, if not twice. It should be complete and satisfactory, without lumpiness.

What are the causes of constipation? Ignoring the calls of nature when they come; not drinking enough water daily to prevent the build-up of poisons; eating the wrong foods; too little physical activity; nervous tension; all of these can and do lead to constipation.

In order to prevent constipation, and reduce your chances of arthritis, you should:

1. Drink plenty of water.

2. Establish regular times for moving your bowels.

3. Get plenty of physical exercise.

4. Eat fruits for breakfast, and for lunch at least one raw vegetable along with a cooked one.

5. Avoid unnecessary tension caused by fear and anxiety.

If arthritis is attached in time, recovery is the general rule, but if the joints are already too far gone, they can never be fully restored. Yet, even then, considerable mobility can be regained and the pain and discomfort drastically reduced by proper nourishment and exercise. Recovery has little to do with the age of the patient. What's more important is the patient's vitality, her constitution and her state of mind. For older people there is also a slower *rate* of recovery.

HOW TO DEAL WITH TENSION AND STRESS

In our civilization we are constantly being subjected to stress and tension of one kind or another. It often seems like there is no escape. Alarm clocks don't go off; cars won't start; buses and trains leave without us; bills come due; bad news assaults us constantly; we get involved in personal arguments, etc. Although we can't avoid them in this day and age, we can do our best to minimize their effects upon us.

Recently, experiments were made on two groups of rats. The only difference between the two groups was that one was subjected to all kinds of stress; kinds that we humans experience every day. The control group was not, but was otherwise the same and observed for the same period.

The test rats were subjected to things like: hunger, fatigue, frustration, too much heat, too much cold, etc. When both groups were autopsied, it was found that in the "stress group" the stomach linings, and the adrenal and thymus glands were gorged with blood, misshapen, diseased and enlarged. In the control group these organs were normal.

Since both groups had been protected against accidental intervention of bacteria, virus, poison or disease, the conclusion was inescapable that the emotions had caused these abnormalities in the rats.

In humans stress has been determined to be involved in upsetting the glandular system and to lead to arthritis, high blood pressure, diabetes, coronaries, ulcers, allergies and kidney trouble. Prolonged tension will increase certain hormone secretions, quicken the pulse and raise the blood pressure.

People who combat fatigue with tranquilizers, "pep" pills and barbiturates are only concealing the problem, not correcting it. They are only postponing a day of reckoning.

We can't avoid stress in this society, but there are many ways we can deal with it and reduce its effects. The first would be to retain a sense of humor about frustrating situations. Use it to sidestep minor irritations and to insulate yourself against petty annoyances.

If you can't joke about your problem, talk it out. Talk it over with a friend or confidant rather than just sitting around stewing about it. Maybe the friend won't even be able to propose a viable solution for you, but somehow just the talking, the putting of the problem into words gives us a broader view of the problem and possibly our own foolishness. If we are in the right, we may still see that we have no need to "make a federal case" out of whatever is bothering us. In short, a friend can help us put it into perspective.

When you feel yourself getting tense over something, relax. Escape. Take little ten minute vacations from problems whenever you can. Foreigners can't understand why we work so hard at everything, including our leisure. They feel we don't know how to pause.

Another suggestion is to take one thing at a time. Sometimes our tension comes from a knowledge of our own limitations as compared with what we feel must be done within a certain time frame. But if you take one element of the problem at a time you will find that having completed that will make you ready to do another and perhaps some of the other things yet to be done will be found capable of being postponed.

If it's anger that's making you tense, work it off. Putter in the garden; cook a surprise for supper; clean the attic or the broom closet; paint that cupboard or do some minor carpentry no one ever gets around to; get involved in a physical sport or take a long walk.

Alternatively listen to some music to calm you down; better yet, if you play an instrument, make your own music. If you don't play, take lessons so that you will be able to release tension in that creative manner.

Once in a while in an argument, give in. If you do, you'll usually find that others will also concede a point or two and before you know it the problem will be well on its way to solution. You will feel more relaxed and you'll have a feeling of satisfaction, whereas if you had stubbornly held out for your point of view, all you would have is tension and bitterness. One way you're helping yourself, one way you're hurting.

Lastly, learn to accept things and people you cannot change. Live and let live. Stand your ground when you believe you are right but do it in a calm manner, allowing for a tactful retreat if you realize you are in error. But some people may be impervious to logical argument; so let them be; why should you get an ulcer over someone else's obstinacy?

To help you soothe your nerves, instead of taking an aspirin or an alcoholic drink, try one of these homemade tonics:

1. Beat an egg to a froth. Add enough grapejuice to fill the glass and mix well in a blender. Drink it slowly so you can savor it all the way down. This drink is rich in amino acids and enzymes and is thus equipped to restore calmness to your tensed-up body and mind.

2. Or, to a well-beaten egg, add honey and two teaspoons of carob powder (from a health store). Blend with a tablespoon of non-fat dry milk powder and a bit of vanilla. Add enough water to fill up a glass and shake it thoroughly. Again, sip it s-l-o-w-l-y.

3. Try heating a cup or two of fresh apple juice just enough to bring it to a simmer, and then remove from the fire. Add 4 table-spoons of apple cider vinegar, two tablespoons of honey (or a "pinch" of cinnamon). Stir vigorously and pour into a tall glass. Savor it slowly and you will find it a dynamo of natural minerals you need to calm your endocrine glands.

If you are fortunate enough to have a good size health-food store near you, you may feel like trying some old-fashioned *herbal tonics*. You can make your elixir from any one of the following herbs, available at many health stores (some in a sort of tea bag):

- Camomile
- Cinchona bark

- Dill
- Peach leaves
- Pennyroyal
- Redclover
- Rosemary
- Sage
- Spearmint
- Thyme
- Valerian
- Wild cherry
- Peppermint

Just take a teaspoonful of the herb and let it steep in a cup of boiled water. Strain out the leaves and sip slowly.

Vitamins, as might be expected, also have a role in relief of stress. When you are under stress, your body uses up in seconds the vitamin C you have stored. You can see that when a person goes through a prolonged emotional crisis her body can be very deficient in vitamin C. And since that is so valuable in resisting infection, she will fall easy prey to colds, infections, arthritis, etc.

Certain foods have been referred to as "natural tranquilizers." Things like vitamin E (in wheat germ), lecithin (in soy beans), and the B-Complex vitamins (in brewer's yeast) are all noted for their soothing effects on the brain and the nerves. Calcium, too, is noted as a painkiller and nerve-soother.

So once again, as you have seen all through this book, the physical and the emotional are intimately involved with the nutritional. Just improving your diet isn't going to do the trick; nor is just adding physical exercise. They all complement each other.

RECOMMENDED FURTHER READING:

"Secrets of Health and Beauty," Linda Clark, 1970, Devin-Adair Company.

"Stay Young Longer," Linda Clark, 1968, Devin-Adair Company.

"Beauty and Health the Scandinavian Way," Gunilla Knutson, 1969, Avon Books.

"Facial Wrinkles," Dr. R. A. Richardson, 1964, Health Research, Mokelumna Hill, Calif.

"Natural Beauty Secrets," Deborah Rutledge, 1966, Avon Books.

"Victory Over Arthritis," Rasmus Alsaker, M. D., 1966, Groton Press.

CHAPTER EIGHT

NATURAL BEAUTY THROUGH YOGA

Only recently yoga was considered a bizzarre fad; now it is widely accepted. One finds it being practiced by film stars, writers, housewives, business executives and students; by young and old alike. What is it doing in a book on Natural Organic Beauty? Simply because it is one of the best means to attain a naturally attractive figure, and it will assist your body to function better on your natural foods diet.

Yoga is over 4,000 years old, yet its principles are as valid today as ever. Modern science has had to admit that yogic exercises, which were designed long before men knew with any accuracy how the internal workings of the body functioned, actually benefit the body in its respiratory and digestive systems, as well as stimulating the blood circulation *in a very scientific manner.*

It is a systematized science of physical conditioning which results in more healthful living. It helps you to bring out your inner beauty by making your body a more healthy and vibrant one. Used in conjunction with a natural diet, you will attain undreamed-of beauty goals.

Developing muscles is recognized by practitioners of yoga as being only one step in physical well-being. True health depends on the integrated functioning of all organs. Yoga helps make this possible by removing conditions which are currently preventing you from being naturally healthy.

The essential difference between yoga and other types of physical exercises (orthodox calisthenics, for instance) is that they operate by forcing the muscles to perform certain movements over and over, quickly and violently. Yoga, however, stresses the slow stretching of particular muscles only to the comfortable limit of your individual body, and then holding them stretched for various brief periods of time.

Yoga is opposed to violent muscle movements because they cause fatigue and a strain on the heart. In yoga, all movements are gradual and slow, with proper breathing tempos, and in a mood of relaxation.

Another result of the fatigue caused by orthodox physical exercises is the production of large quantities of lactic acid. When muscles contract, the glycogen in the body breaks down into lactic acid so that additional energy can be released. When too much lactic acid accumulates, the muscles become temporarily unable to contract. Stretching a muscle before it contracts (as in yoga) enables it to contract more forcibly.

Fatigue is a result of the inability of the muscles to get enough oxygen to oxidize a sufficient amount of the lactic acid formed.

The main objective of any exercise (by itself) is to increase the circulation of the blood and the intake of oxygen. This can be achieved by relatively simple movements of the spine and various joints of the body, during deep breathing, yet without violent movement of the muscles.

There is nothing strenuous about yoga. Perhaps you have seen pictures of Indians who have contorted themselves into all kinds of imaginable shapes. These are not what we are suggesting in this book; these are for more advanced students of yoga. But it should be remembered that even *these* unusual contortions of the body can be achieved without great strain, after practice.

In all yoga exercises the movements are performed slowly, with grace and with ease. Instead of aching muscles afterward produced by ordinary exercise, you will feel a genuine "refreshment" of body and spirit. This will soon be transferred to your outward appearance.

The principal cause of the stiffness and inflexibility of our bodies comes from tension. We are tense due to problems brought on by interpersonal relations, job worries, worries about the future, social pressures and the million and one pressures of urban life among cars, factories, and airplanes.

In western civilization, particularly in America, the average person of 30 is almost as stiff and inelastic as is a person 60 years old. Through yoga, tension is eased without resorting to the aid of tranquilizers. Your skin tone will quickly improve, and those bodies grown flabby with neglect and disuse will take on a renewed resilience.

Aside from making you feel better and more relaxed, moderate and consistent yoga exercises will help your body to become more capable of meeting the demands you place upon it. Other benefits from the proper application of yoga include elimination of toxins accumulated in the body and retaining the elasticity of the arteries, thus preventing heart disease.

In preparing for your daily session of yoga exercises, it is well to set the proper mood. You will naturally want to find a quiet room and quiet time of day, and a maximum of privacy. It should also be a well-ventilated area and one which gives you a feeling of calm (such as a bedroom). Make sure you have a firm surface (not a bed or heavy foam mattress) but not something rock-hard (like tile or cement). Don't forget to take the phone off the hook, also.

Be sure to wear comfortable clothes in which you can move easily.

Now we begin a description of various yoga exercises which benefit a specific area of the body.

ABDOMEN

The Abdominal Contraction

Stand with your feet slightly apart and bend your knees until you are in a one-quarter squat. Place your palms on your thighs, fingers pointed toward each other, about halfway from your groin to your knee. Shift most of your weight onto your arms, giving you a free feeling in your abdomen.

From this position, exhale all the air out of the lungs through your mouth. Do NOT INHALE while performing the rest of the exercise. Now suck your abdomen in and upward into your chest, creating a hollow indentation in your abdomen, and hold for the count of "one."

Now pop your abdomen back out with a vigorous but not violent movement. Do this in and out movement five times on a single exhaling of the breath. Then stand up erect and inhale. Wait until your breath returns to normal before resuming.

Benefits from the Abdominal Contraction:

1. Relieves constipation.

2. Strengthens abdominal muscles.

3. Aids in reducing weight around the waist.

4. Helps restore a dropped abdomen to proper place.

The Triangle Pose

Stand erect keeping the feet about 2 or 3 feet apart. Bring the arms to shoulder height, palms down and bend to the left slowly. Touch the left toes with the left hand and remain for 5 seconds before returning to the standing position. Repeat to the right. Repeat four times.

Benefits from the Triangle Pose:

1. Strengthens abdominal muscles and spine muscles.

2. Reduces abdominal fat tissue.

WAIST

The Side Bends

Stand erect, with hands at your sides and feet slightly apart (about the distance from one shoulder to the other). Raise your arms slowly out from your sides until they are extended sideways at shoulder level. Bend slowly to your right side, taking at least 10 seconds to reach the farthest limit of your position. Hold there for 10 seconds. Straighten up slowly to the erect position, and then lower your arms slowly to your sides. Repeat for the left side. Do three on each side.

Benefits from side bends:

1. Reduces weight in the waist.

2. Tones up seldom-used muscles in the thighs.

3. Removes tension.

4. Strengthens relatively weak muscles in the sides.

5. Gives the spine a sideways stretch.

Alternate Leg-Pull

From a seated position with your legs extended straight in front of you (toes and heels together) and your back erect, bend your left leg at the knee until it brings your left foot close enough for you to grasp it with both hands (without bending the back). Place the sole of your left foot against the inside of your right thigh. Your heel should be as close to your groin as you can get it without strain.

Now slowly raise both arms straight out in front of you until you have them extended at eye level, palms down. Without bending your elbows, cross your left arm over your right arm and bend forward slowly. Twist your body slowly forward so that the right side of your head (and face) will be facing the right leg (still extended). Attempt to grasp the outside of the right leg at any point you can reach.

If you can't reach the leg with your left hand, simply reach toward it as far as is comfortable. Either way, hold your farthest position for 10 seconds.

Go very slowly in coming out of this posture, going limp all over and twisting yourself back to the erect sitting pose as you slide your hand along your thigh, back to the starting position. Straighten your left leg back out again, also slowly. Repeat to the right side.

Benefits from alternate leg-pulls:

1. Trims excess weight from the waist.

2. Restores limberness to the legs.

3. Helps reduce hips and thighs.

4. Replaces tension in the back with new flexibility.

5. Limbers up the spinal column.

HIPS

The Half Locust

Lying on your abdomen with your hands at your sides, rest your face on one cheek. Keep your toes together and go completely limp. Bring your heels together, with toes extended outward from the body. Clench your hands into fists and place them thumbs down against your sides. Now turn your head and rest your chin on the floor.

Raise your left leg as high in the air as you can. Pushing downward with your fists will help to raise the leg even higher than you otherwise could. Keep the upraised knee straight and hold for 10 seconds. Slowly lower your leg, using at least 10 more seconds to do so. Breathe normally throughout the exercise.

Rest limply for a few moments and then repeat with the right leg.

Benefits from the half locust:

1. Firms and strengthens hips, buttocks and thighs.

2. Aids in reducing hips, buttocks and thighs.

3. Strengthens muscles of the abdomen and lower back.

4. Tones seldom-used muscles of the pelvic region.

THIGHS

The Knee and Thigh Stretch

Start in a seated position with your legs stretched out in front of you—knees straight, toes and heels together. Bending both legs at the knees, bring them toward you, heels still together) until the soles of your feet come together with the heels against your groin. Clasp your hands around both your feet, with fingers intertwined (as in prayer).

Still sitting erectly and holding your feet, press your knees down as close to the floor as possible by flexing the thigh muscles and bearing down. Hold this pose for 10 seconds. Slowly come out of it by gently releasing the pressure on your legs and allowing the knees to rise to the original position. Relax and then repeat the exercise.

Benefits from the knee and thigh stretch:

1. Removes tension from the thighs.

2. Stretches the seldom-used muscles and tendons of the inner thighs.

3. Aids in trimming weight from the thighs.

4. Increases bounce and vigor in your walk.

The Spread Leg Stretch

Sit erect with your legs extended straight out in front of you, toes and heels together. Without bending your knees, spread your legs as far apart as you can. Then place one hand on the top of each thigh, as far away from you as possible without bending forward.

Now slide your hands forward down your legs slowly as you lean forward to extend your reach. Only stretch as far as you can without strain. When you can reach no further, grasp with your hands whatever part of your legs they have reached.

Close your eyes and hold the posture motionless for 10 seconds. Then straighten your elbows and, releasing your grip, allow your hands to slide back up your thighs as you slowly straighten your spine. Your head should be the last part of you to return to the upright position. Rest and then repeat two times.

Benefits of the Spread Leg Stretch:

1. The legs are stretched, limbered, firmed up and relieved from tension.

2. Helps trim excessive weight from the thighs.

3. Removes flabbiness from the thighs.

4. Limbers back and spine.

5. Improves circulation.

6. General relaxation of the body.

LEGS

The Standing Twist

Stand erect and pull in your abdomen and hold your chest high. Imagine yourself hanging by a cable coming out of the top of your head, with your feet just touching the floor enough to carry your weight. Heels together; toes slightly apart.

Raise your arms straight in front of you (elbows locked) until they are straight out at eye level, thumbs touching each other. Slowly inhale one breath as you bring the arms up. Go back to normal breathing when arms are in front of you. Also rise slowly on your toes as the arms arise.

Keeping thumbs together, begin moving your arms toward the right, turning only your upper torso. Turn as far to the right as you comfortably can, keeping your eyes on the meeting place of the two thumbs. Hold for ten seconds. Then slowly return to the facing-forward position. Slowly come down from tiptoes as you lower your arms until you are in the starting position again. Repeat to the left.

Benefits of the Standing Twist:

1. Strengthens legs by stretching muscles and tissues of the legs in a spiral manner.

2. Helps reduce the waist.

3. Spine is also twisted in a spiral manner and its flexibility is restored.

THE NECK

The Neck Stretch

Lying on your abdomen, and resting on your elbows, cup your head in your hands by placing your fingers along your temples and your wrists almost touching under your chin. Turn your head to the left so that your chin rests in your left hand and the back of your head rests in your right.

Slowly turn your head even further to the left as far as it can go without strain and with only the most gentle help from your hands. Hold this stretch for five seconds and then slowly do a complete reversal to the right as far as you can go. Do this three times to each side.

Benefits from the neck stretch:

1. Relieves tension in the neck.

2. Loosens and limbers-up a stiff neck.

3. Relieves pain in the neck.

The Slow Neck Roll

Drop your head very slowly by letting your neck go limp until your head hangs forward onto your chest, then very slowly roll your head around to your right side. Keep your neck limp and let the weight of your head pull on your neck muscles.

Continue rolling the head very slowly until it is hanging backward. From there you continue to roll, this time to the left until you have made a complete circle. Reverse direction and repeat three times in each direction.

Benefits from the slow neck roll:

1. Irons out tension lines.

2. Relieves pains in the neck.

3. Removes tension from the neck.

ARMS

The Backward Stretch

Assume a sitting position, with feet stretched out in front of you, heels together, hands palms down on the floor at your sides. Keeping elbows straight and heels on the floor begin to push your torso slowly off the floor. Slide your heels slightly forward in order to straighten your body. If your palms are facing toward the rear, your whole body should form a perfect triangle, defined by your body, your arms and the floor. Slowly tilt your head back and hold for a few seconds.

To return from this position, slowly lower your buttocks to the floor while holding arms and knees straight. Repeat two or three times.

Benefits from the backward stretch:

1. Strengthens arms.

2. Firms up the abdomen.

3. Helps release tension in the spine.

ANKLES

The Simple Posture

Sit cross-legged on the floor, with each foot resting under the calf of the other leg.

Benefits of the simple posture:

1. Increases circulation in the legs.

2. Loosens ankle, knee and hip joints.

3. Relaxes the nerves and the mind.

4. Introductory step to the "Lotus Position."

The Half Lotus

Assume a seated position with your legs straight out in front of you, heels and toes together. Bending your left leg at the knee, bring that foot up toward your body so you can grasp it with your hands. Your left knee should remain as close to the floor as comfortable.

Place the sole of your left foot against the inside of your right thigh, drawing your left heel up as closely as you can to your groin.

Do the same with your right foot, except that as it nears your body, lift the right foot with your hands and place the outside of it at the point where your body meets your left thigh. The sole of your right foot should face upward as far as is comfortable. Rest your wrists on the forward edges of your knees, palms down.

This is the famous Half Lotus Position. The Full Lotus Position is only for very advanced yoga students. Why? It involves crossing your feet in this manner while standing on your head!

Benefits from the half lotus:

1. Removes stiffness from ankles, knees and hip joints.

2. Improves circulation in those areas.

3. A condition of physical balance is achieved.

4. Banishes tension from the legs.

BACK

Complete Leg and Back Stretch

Sit with legs extended in front of you, toes and heels together; knees straight; back erect. Raise your arms until they are straight in front of you at eye level; thumbs together, palms down.

Bend slightly backward from the waist and then bend slowly forward. Aim your hands for the farthest part of your legs that you can comfortably reach. Take at least ten seconds to get there and then grasp firmly whatever part of your ankle, calf, knee or thigh that you can reach.

Now very gently bend your elbows outward and pull yourself (your head and upper body) downward. Ultimately you want to place your nose between your knees while your fingers grasp your toes and your elbows rest on the floor. That of course is the ultimate. The great thing about yoga is that you also can obtain great benefits from any way station position you can reach.

Close your eyes and let your neck go limp. Breathe normally and hold motionless for ten seconds. Then straighten your elbows and slide your hands back up your thighs until you are in an upright sitting position again. Let your head be the last part of you to straighten up.

Benefits from the leg and back stretch:

1. Gives full elasticity to the spine when bending forward.

2. Removes deep tension throughout the spine and back.

3. Develops and tones up the muscles in the back.

4. Stretches tendons behind the knees, returning elasticity to the legs.

5. Helps reduce weight in the hips, abdomen and back.

THE SPINE

The Cobra

This exercise is superficially similar to the "push-ups" we all learned in gym class, but it is very different and much more beneficial.

Lie on your abdomen with your hands at your sides, palms upward, with your head resting on one cheek. Let your body go limp all over. Slowly turn your head until you are resting on your forehead and nose.

Slowly raise your head and back. When your head will not go back further, continue raising your trunk. Let your eyes look toward the top of your head as it moves backward. Your arms should be used to push your trunk to its comfortable limit with your elbows straight. Do not allow your pelvic area to leave the ground. (This is one place there is an obvious difference with a pushup.)

When you have reached your own limit, hold for ten seconds and then begin coming down by bending your elbows gradually and dropping your trunk an inch or so at a time. First your stomach will touch down, then your diaphragm and then your chest. Finally lower your head and bring arms slowly back to their original position. Turn your face to return to the position of resting on your cheek. Rest several moments before repeating.

Benefits from the cobra:

1. Stretches every vertebra in your spinal column from the base of the spine to your neck.

2. Restores limberness to entire back and spine.

3. Helpful in dispelling fatigue.

4. Revitalizing to the entire body.

5. Improves posture.

6. Develops muscles of the chest and bust.

7. Strengthens back muscles.

8. Firms hips and reduces buttocks.

CHEST

Chest Expansion Posture

Stand erect with hands at your sides and heels several inches apart. Raise your arms slowly in front of you, elbows straight, until your hands are touching each other at shoulder level with palms down. Then, with your elbows straight, bring your arms back around you as if you were doing a swimmer's breast stroke, and clasp your hands behind you. You may have to lower them somewhat at first in order to reach, but then straighten them back up as far as is comfortable.

Now bend slowly back at the waist, keeping your knees straight. Let your head drop back with your neck limp so that you are looking upward at the ceiling, bending only so far as is comfortable, and hold for 5 seconds. Straighten up slowly and, without stopping, bend slowly forward until your head is as far down to the floor as you can get without discomfort. Ultimately, you want your forehead to reach your knees.

Hold for 10 seconds, then slowly straighten up erect. Relax while standing, and then repeat three times.

Benefits from the chest expansion posture:

1. Develops the chest and firms the bust muscles.

2. Improves the posture.

3. Promotes flexibility of the spine in both directions.

4. Relieves tension throughout the body.

5. Trims a flabby abdomen.

6. Improves circulation in the head.

7. Strengthens seldom-used shoulder muscles.

SHOULDERS

The Shoulder Stand

Lie on your back with your hands at your sides and let your body go limp. Your hands should be flush with your body, palms down on the floor. Press downward on the floor with your hands and begin to slowly lift your legs off the floor, keeping your knees straight.

Slowly raise your legs until you have them straight up in the air at a ninety degree angle to the rest of your body. The slower you do this part of the exercise, the stronger you will make your abdomen. Now increase the pressure of your hands against the floor and call into play the muscles in your back and abdomen, and raise your buttocks and lower back off the floor completely. Tilt your legs toward your head to retain your balance.

Place your left hand against the kidney region of your back and brace up your lower back area with it. Do the same with the right hand and now extend your feet as straight up into the air as you can. The effect should be a sort of modified "headstand." Instead of supporting your body by standing on your head, you are supporting it with your shoulders. Try to hold this position for one minute.

To come down from the position, first bend your knees and bring them down until the knees are an inch or two above your nose. Return your hands to the floor, palms down. Now unroll your trunk back onto the floor, *slowly*. Now bring your legs back up until they are perpendicular again and then lower them straight down to the floor (knees straight at all times). Go completely limp and rest for at least 2 minutes.

Benefits from the shoulder stand:

1. Stimulates circulation all through the body.

2. Stimulates the brain (as a result of the increased blood circulation) and improves mental faculties.

3. Benefits the hair by increasing circulation to the scalp.

4. Aids in reducing excess weight.

5. Counteracts the sagging of abdominal muscles and organs.

6. Relieves varicose veins.

7. Helps the complexion by circulating blood through facial tissues.

8. Produces a deep overall body relaxation.

EYES

Three Eye Movements

1. From a sitting position in which you are comfortable, look ahead and visualize a large clockface. Look at the imaginery number 12 at the "top" of this clock. Quickly focus on the other

numbers in succession, rolling your eyes in a clockwise motion without moving your head. When you reach twelve again, do the same thing in a *counter* clockwise motion. Close your eyes and rest them for 30 seconds before repeating.

2. Do the same thing with your eyes closed or covered.

3. Hold your index finger up in front of your face about six inches from your eyes. Focus on the tip of the finger or upon the fingernail. Don't allow it to waver, and don't look at anything else. After about three seconds look beyond the finger to the most distant object you can see. If you are outdoors you are in the best place for this exercise. Make your eyes focus on the hill or tree or building and hold that for 3 seconds. Then focus back on your finger tip. Continue alternating for ten times.

Benefits from the eye exercises:

1. Relieves tension in the eyes, makes them look alive again.

2. Deeply relaxing to entire nervous system.

3. Relieves eye fatigue immediately.

4. Strengthens eye muscles and may possibly save you from having to get glasses (or stronger ones if you already have them).

BREATH CONTROL

The Cleansing Breath

Sit erect in a cross-legged position and inhale about a third of a lungful of air through the nose while expanding the abdomen as far as it can go.

With a single sudden and vigorous movement, pull your abdomen in as swiftly as you can. At the same time, vigorously expel all the air in the lungs through your nostrils. The effect should seem to be that you were punched in the stomach and the air was forced out of your nose as a reaction.

Permit your abdomen to expand again so that the air is sucked back into your lungs through your nostrils. Now repeat. Ten of these is a complete breath exercise.

Benefits from the Cleansing Breath:

1. Cleanses lung tissue of impurities.

2. Relieves symptoms of colds and other respiratory ailments.

3. Relieves sinuses and clogged nasal passages.

4. Strengthens abdominal wall.

5. Strengthens and develops diaphragm.

6. Strengthens the lungs.

The Complete Breath

Sit cross-legged on the floor. Prepare for this exercise by pulling in your abdomen and at the same time exhaling through your nose until your lungs are empty. Now inhale slowly, smoothly and quietly through your nose, pushing out your abdomen as far as you can. This should take about 5 seconds.

Continuing to inhale slowly through your nose, pull in your abdomen slowly and expand your chest. This should take another 5 seconds. Raise your shoulders slightly and hold the breath for 5 seconds.

Exhale through the nose, relaxing your chest and shoulders as you do. Don't relax your abdomen; keep that pulled in firmly throughout the entire holding and exhalation of breath. Take 10 seconds to exhale. Do three complete breaths at a time.

1. Develops and expands the entire chest.

2. Increases the clarity of the mind.

3. Develops the diaphragm.

4. Purifies the blood by the increased oxygen intake.

5. Increases resistance to colds.

6. Strengthens and calms the nervous system.

THE ART OF RELAXATION

Recharging Technique

Lie on your back as limp as you can be, with your legs slightly apart. Your arms should be at your side about a foot or so from your body, with the palms up. Raise your left leg a few inches and let it fall (plop!) back to the floor of its own weight. Do the same with your right leg.

Bend your left arm at the elbow so that you raise your hand and forearm (while keeping the upper arm on the floor). Then let the hand fall as you did the legs. Repeat with the right forearm, then the entire left arm and the entire right arm.

Using as little physical effort as possible, lift your pelvis and buttocks area off the floor slightly and allow it to fall limply back down. Lastly, do the same with your abdomen. Remain motionless in the original position for a few moments.

Mentally order your *toes* to go limp. This may take a great deal of concentration but you will catch on soon. Then do the same with your feet. Wait a while and concentrate on your ankles, until you can make them relax. Continue all the way up your body, section by section, until you are relaxed all the way to your neck.

Very slowly (take about 15 seconds) roll your head to the right. Then roll your head slowly to the left, taking 30 seconds to do it. Roll your head slowly back to the right—again taking a half minute. Now tell your neck to go limp. Lie there with your eyes closed commanding each part of your face to become limp in succession. Lie there for perhaps three minutes in this state of relaxation, breathing long, calm breaths from your abdomen.

These exercises can be practiced either morning or afternoon with considerable benefits to you, but do not exceed about one hour at one session. And always remember not to strain or force any muscles beyond the comfortable limit. You will find that this limit expands as you strengthen your body through the exercises. Remember, too, to breathe deeply and work out in a well-ventilated room.

RECOMMENDED FURTHER READING:

"Yoga for Beauty and Health," Eugene Rawls and Eve Diskin, 1967, Parker Publishing Company.

"The Complete Illustrated Book of Yoga," Swami Vishnudevananda, 1960, The Julian Press Inc.

CHAPTER NINE

TASTY, YET HEALTHFUL EATING

Breakfasts

French Toast

½ cup fresh milk
½ cup powdered milk
2 to 4 eggs
1 tsp. salt
6 or 8 slices stale whole wheat bread

Mix the milks together and beat until smooth, add the eggs and beat slightly. Soak the bread in the mixture, and then saute slowly in partially hardened margarine. Soak until browned on both sides. Serve with apple sauce or fresh, crushed and sweetened berries.

Omelet

1 egg
1 tbsp. water
2 tsp. mineral salt
1 tbsp. apricot-kernel oil

Beat the egg well, adding water and salt while continuing to beat. Add yogurt and blend well. Heat the skillet and add oil, then the omelet. Cover with a lid and cook slowly over a low heat. With a pancake turner, lift the edges and tilt the pan so the uncooked butter will run to the bottom. When the top is set, fold the omelet in the middle with a spatula and turn off the heat. Add a few slices of cheese to the top and let them melt under the lid. Serve hot.

Cornmeal Mush With Fruit

1 cup cornmeal
2 cups cold water
½ cup dried apricots (mashed)
1 cup of prunes (cooked, pitted, mashed)
½ cup applesauce
½ cup banana (mashed)

Place cornmeal in salted water over fire and stir frequently until it comes to a rolling boil. Cover with a tight lid and turn off heat. Let stand for 20 minutes and then add one of above fruits. Use a different one each day.

Thin Pancakes

¼ cup whole wheat pastry flour

1 tsp. salt

⅓ cup powdered milk

1 cup fresh milk

4 eggs

Sift the flour, salt and milk together and then add the eggs and fresh milk, beating well. Heat a large frying pan and brush it with a generous amount of partially hardened margarine. Take about a fourth of the batter and drop into pan, creating 3 pancakes. Saute until light brown on both sides. Place them on a hot plate and repeat for rest of the batter. Serve with grated cheese, applesauce, or fresh sweetened berries.

Swedish Muesli

4 tbsp. rolled oats

4 tbsp. lemon juice

¼ lb. chopped nuts

2 bananas

2 large eating apples

2 oz. brown sugar

1 small container yogurt

Peel, core and chop the apples. Peel and slice the banana. Mix all ingredients together.

Whole Buckwheat Groats

1 cup whole buckwheat groats

2 cups water

1 tsp. Spike (vegetable salt)

2 tbsp. safflower oil

Heat the oil in a heavy skillet. Stir in the groats mixed with the beaten egg. Add salt and brown slightly, keeping it stirred with a spoon. Then add the water and bring to a boil. Reduce heat, cover tightly and let simmer until all the liquid is absorbed.

Millet Hulled

½ cup hulled millet
1 cup water
1 cup milk
1 tbsp. honey
½ tsp. Spike
dried apricots, soaked overnight

Heat water and milk in the top of a double boiler. Add millet and steam over boiling water until millet is tender (about 30 minutes). Add dried apricots and honey.

Salads

Beauty Salad

1 head of lettuce (chopped up)
4 Jerusalem artichokes
2 tomatoes
1 cup alfalfa sprouts
1 avocado
3 stalks diced celery
1 green pepper (shredded)
3 carrots (shredded)

Mix well in a salad bowl. Blend with your favorite salad dressing and top with slices of tomatoes, avocado and alfalfa sprouts.

Green Pea Salad

1 cup fresh green peas
2 stalks crisp green celery
1 small bunch of green scallions
1 green pepper
2 small tomatoes

Dice up the celery stalks, celery heart, scallions, pepper and tomatoes. Mix with peas and serve on lettuce with your favorite dressing.

Potato Salad

3 potatoes (steamed or boiled)
1 small bunch of green onions (chopped)
1 cup chopped celery
2 tsp. celery seed
¾ tsp. salt

¼ cup chopped parsley
2 hard-boiled eggs (sliced)

Peel and cube the cooked potatoes. Mix ingredients with a dressing made up of:

½ cup yogurt
1 tsp. honey
1 tsp. lemon juice

German Potato Salad

1 large potato for each person
1 pickled gherkin per person
1 tbsp. olive oil per person
1 tsp. tarragon vinegar per person
   chopped parsley
   salt
   black pepper

Boil potatoes in their skins until tender. Allow to cool and then peel and dice them small. Dress them with oil and then vinegar. Dice the gherkins and mix with potatoes. Sprinkle with salt and plenty of black pepper. Garnish with chopped parsley.

Tossed Summer Salad

4 sliced tomatoes
2 diced green peppers
2 cups diced cucumbers
1 Bermuda onion, chopped
2 diced hearts & tops of celery
3 tbsp. mixed fresh herbs, minced

Toss all ingredients lightly and then moisten with yogurt.

Tossed Winter Salad

3 cups cooked lima beans
3 tbsp. oil
1 lemon (juice and rind)
3 tbsp. minced parsley
1 tbsp. minced dill
4 sliced scallions
1 hard cooked egg, sliced
1 tomato, sliced
1 green pepper, minced

Toss all ingredients lightly. Serve cold.

Cole Slaw

4 cups finely shredded cabbage
1 cup finely shredded carrots
¼ cup finely chopped green peppers
¼ cup honey
1 cup yogurt
¼ tsp. salt
2 tsp. celery salt

Mix together and chill before serving.

Classic Caesar Salad

3 garlic cloves (chopped)
1 cup olive oil
2 cups whole wheat bread crumb cubes
½ cup grated Parmesan cheese
½ cup crumbled blue cheese
1 tbsp. Worcestershire sauce
½ tsp. dry mustard
1 tsp. salt
½ tsp. pepper
2 eggs
½ cup lemon juice

Mix chopped garlic cloves into olive oil and let stand several hours at room temperature. Toast bread crumb cubes in oven until brown and crisp. Pour above ingredients over 3 qts. of crisp greens of your choice, breaking the eggs just before adding the lemon juice. Serve at once while crumbs are still crunchy.

Soybean-Cheese Salad

2 cups cooked soybeans
2 cups cooked, diced vegetables
½ cup grated cheese

Toss all ingredients and moisten with yogurt.

Salad of India

6 sliced bananas
3 tbsp. minced mint
½ cup dates, pitted and chopped
½ cup nuts, ground

Arrange a bed of greens and place bananas on them. Sprinkle rest of ingredients on.

Cucumbers in Sour Cream

2 cucumbers, thinly sliced
3 tbsp. chopped chives
1 cup sour cream
3 tbsp. lemon juice
½ tsp. powdered dill

Mix lemon juice into sour cream. Mix cucumbers with chives. Stir in the dill and dressing. Salt and pepper to taste. Serve chilled.

Tomato Salad

1 lb. firm tomatoes
½ cup minced onions
½ cup corn oil
   fresh dill
   white vinegar (to taste)
   sweet basil leaves
   salt and pepper

Slice the tomatoes nice and thick and mix with minced onion, dill and sweet basil. Toss in the oil until coated, then add vinegar. Season with salt and black pepper and toss again. Chill slightly before serving.

Tomato-Avocado Salad

2 stalks diced celery
1 chopped green pepper
1 chopped onion
1 avocado, peeled and mashed
4 tomatoes
1 lemon (for juice)
2 tbsp. honey

Mix celery, pepper and onion and add avocado. Scoop out tomato pulp, cut fine and add to mixture. Add juice of the lemon. Fill tomatoes and serve with yogurt.

Green and Red Pepper Salad

   green peppers
   red peppers
1 large onion, minced
   corn oil
   lemon juice
   salt
   black pepper

Scald both peppers in boiling water and plunge them into cold. Remove stalks, together with all seeds and pith inside. Slice the peppers very thin. Mix other ingredients together and add the peppers. Allow to cool before serving.

Eggplant Salad

1 raw eggplant, diced
  cider vinegar
½ tsp. basil
½ tsp. parsley, minced
1 onion, sliced
1 bunch water cress
2 hard-cooked eggs, quartered
  ripe olives

Marinate the eggplant in vinegar with herbs and onion for two hours. Toss with the watercress. Garnish with eggs and olives. Serve with dressing of your choice.

Tuna Salad

1 cup tuna flakes
2 hard-cooked eggs
½ cup finely chopped celery
½ cup cooked peas
½ tsp. salt
¼ cup minced parsley
½ tsp. paprika

Mix ingredients together lightly, using one chopped egg. Slice the other egg for a topping. Serve on crisp salad greens.

Raw Spinach Salad

1 cup raw spinach
4 ripe tomatoes
2 small onions

Cut up and mix together. Serve on green lettuce leaves. Use lemon juice as a dressing.

Chicory Salad

4 firm heads of chicory
1 head celery
1 large cooking apple
1 medium-size onion

1 raw baby beet
1 cup grated Parmesan cheese
  watercress
  vinegar
  salad oil

Peel and shred vegetables and apple. Separate chicory into leaves. Season with salt and pepper and toss in salad oil. Chill well and serve on bed of watercress, sprinkled with Parmesan.

Yam-Fruit Salad

5 yams, cooked and diced
4 bananas, sliced
3 apples with skins, diced
1 cup seedless grapes

Toss all ingredients lightly. Moisten with favorite dressing.

Cauliflower Salad

½ head uncooked cauliflower
½ cup finely chopped green pepper
½ cup finely chopped celery
1 tsp. salt
½ large head lettuce

Remove outer leaves of cauliflower and cut into paper-thin slices. Mix with pepper, celery and salt. Break lettuce into small pieces and toss into mixture. Top servings with minced parsley.

Greek Cabbage Salad

½ lb. finely shredded white cabbage
1 small shredded raw beet
1 doz. black olives
½ tsp. capers
8 tbsp. red wine vinegar
4 tbsp. olive oil
1 tsp. (heaping) prepared mustard
1 garlic clove (crushed)

Mix cabbage, beets olives, and capers together. Make a dressing of the remainder. Mix together, chill and serve.

Radish-Onion Salad

4 radishes sliced thin
2 green onions sliced thin

¼ cucumber sliced thin
1 cup sprouts
½ cup cottage cheese
½ cup yogurt

Mix vegetables and sprouts and combine with the cheese mixture. Moisten with yogurt.

Fruit Salad

cantaloupe balls
berries
seedless grapes
sliced oranges

Serve on salad greens and sprinkle with shredded coconut and nuts. Use a yogurt dressing.

Date-Carrot Salad

½ cup chopped firm dates
1 cup finely shredded raw carrots
½ cup finely chopped celery
¼ cup yogurt
½ cup chopped nuts
¼ tsp. salt
dash of paprika

Combine and chill. Serve on lettuce.

Meat Dishes

Roast Leg of Lamb

Sprinkle 5 lb. leg of lamb with salt. Place fat side up in open roaster. Make several slits about ½ inch wide and insert slices of garlic and sprinkle with papaya powder. Rub with the juice of one lemon. Roast at 250 degrees, cutting down to 175 later. Baste frequently with the following:

1 tsp. rosemary
1 tsp. thyme
1 tsp. savory
1 tsp. sweet basil
1 tsp. marjoram
½ cup dry white wine

Roasting time should be 1½ hours for rare, 2 hours for medium and 2½ for well done. However, if lamb is not at room temperature when you are ready to roast, add a half hour more.

Lamb and Parsley Stew

3 tbsp. oil
3 large bunches of parsley, minced
10 chopped scallions
2 lbs. lean, cubed, lamb
2 lemons (for juice)
3 tbsp. nutritional yeast
2 cups cooked kidney beans

Heat the oil in a pot. Saute the parsley, scallions and lamb. Add lemon juice and yeast and blend. Cover and let simmer until meat is tender. Then add beans and cook until they are heated thoroughly.

Stuffed Green Peppers

1 cup cooked lima beans
  chopped green beans
  chopped celery
  corn
  diced carrots
½ cup moistened bread crumbs
½ cup grated cheddar cheese
1 green pepper for each person

Remove inside seeds and fibers from green peppers by either slicing off tops or cutting in half lengthwise. Drop into boiling water. Remove from fire and let stand ten or fifteen minutes and drain. Fill the peppers with the mix and cover with buttered crumbs or grated cheese. Set peppers in a shallow pan half-filled with water. Bake in moderate oven for 30 minutes.

Lamb Stew

1½ lbs. lamb shoulder
1 tbsp. salad oil
½ cup chopped celery
½ cup minced parsley
2 tsp. salt
½ tsp. rosemary
½ tsp. ginger
1 doz. small onions, peeled
4 small carrots
¼ cup flour & ¼ cup water, mixed

Cut meat into 1½ inch pieces and brown in salad oil. Add

chopped celery, parsley, salt, rosemary, ginger, onions and carrots to 4 cups of water. Cover and let simmer for an hour.

Kidney Hash

2 tbsp. oil
2 onions sliced
2 cups, cooked, ground kidney
½ tsp. salt
2 tbsp. nutritional yeast
1 cup potatoes, cooked and cubed
½ tsp. thyme
1 tbsp. minced parsley
½ cup roasted, ground soybeans

Heat the oil and saute the onions. Then blend with the remaining ingredients. Pack mixture into an oiled baking dish and bake in a 300 F. oven for 20 minutes.

Ham Casserole

2 cups cooked, ground ham
2 cups cooked corn
1 tsp. salt
3 tbsp. nutritional yeast
1 tbsp. oil
¼ tsp. ground mace
3 tbsp honey
½ cup stock

Spread half the ham in the bottom of an oiled casserole. Mix the ingredients (except the stock) and pour over the ham. Place rest of the ham on top of the mixture, and pour on the stock. Bake in a 300 degree oven for 40 minutes.

Carrot Meat Loaf

2 cups cooked mashed carrots
1 lb. ground beef
1 egg, beaten
½ cup soft whole wheat crumbs
1 small onion, minced
2 tsp. salt
¼ tsp. pepper

Mix thoroughly and bake in greased loaf pan for an hour at 350 degrees.

Braised Liver

1½ lbs. sliced liver
    whole wheat flour
  3 tbsp. oil
  3 tbsp. nutritional yeast
  1 tbsp. minced parsley
  ½ cup cubed carrots
  ½ cup chopped celery
  1 chopped onion
  1 chopped green pepper
  ¼ cup stock

Dredge the liver in the flour. Heat the oil and brown the liver. Then add the remaining ingredients and cover. Continue cooking on top of the stove over a low heat for 20 minutes.

Broiled Liverburgers

1½ lbs. liver, cubed
    stock
  3 onions, chopped
  1 egg
  ½ tsp. oregano
  3 tbsp. parsley
  ½ tsp. salt
  3 tbsp. nutritional yeast

Cook the liver, stock and onions in a covered pan until the liver is soft. Drain. Puree in the blender with the rest of ingredients. Make 12 patties and broil for a few minutes on each side.

Korean Broiled Beef

2 lbs. beef steak, cut into think strips
2 tbsp. oil
3 tbsp. essence of sweet herbs
2 green onions, sliced
1 clove garlic, minced
½ cup stock
½ cup sesame seeds, toasted

Marinate beef in a mixture of remaining ingredients, except sesame seeds, overnight. Remove from the marinade and broil. Garnish with the seeds.

Mock Duck

½ lb. cooked soya beans
½ lb. cooked lentils
1 small onion, chopped
1 cup mashed potatoes
   sweet basil leaves
3 tbsp. butter
2 tbsp. chopped parsley
½ tsp. sage
   tomato juice (to taste)
   salt and pepper

Soak the beans overnight in cold water and then boil them with a teaspoon of salt and a little raw sugar until tender. If you use a pressure cooker, it will take a half hour; otherwise 2 to 4 hours. Add the cooked soya beans to the lentils and the mashed potatoes. Fry the onion in half the butter and add the soya beans to the mixture. Add sage and parsley and season to taste. Shape into tennis-size balls, and put the "ducks" onto a greased baking tin. Pour the rest of the butter (melted) over the ducks and make in a fairly hot oven until deep brown. Serve in a tureen with lots of hot thickened tomato juice.

Liver Kidney Kebab

½ lb. liver, cubed
½ lb. lamb kidney, cubed
½ lb. lamb
3 tomatoes cut in wedges
3 onions, sliced
½ lb. mushrooms
3 tbsp. oil
1 clove garlic, minced

Place on skewers, alternating ingredients. Brush combined oil and garlic over them. Broil, turning frequently.

Potted Calf's Liver

1½ lbs. calf's liver
1 onion, chopped
1 clove garlic, chopped
2 tbsp. celery, chopped
2 tbsp. parsley, minced
1 tsp. salt
1 tbsp. soy flour

    3 tbsp. nutritional yeast
    ½ tsp. basil
    2 tbsp. whole wheat flour
    3 tbsp. oil
    1 cup stock

Cut the slice of liver into 6 pockets, about an inch wide from the top to the bottom. Mix onion, garlic, celery, parsley, salt, soy flour, yeast and basil together, and fill these pockets with the resulting mixture. Tie a string around the liver to keep the filling in place. Dredge the liver in flour. Heat the oil and saute the liver. Add stock and cover the pot. Let simmer for 20 minutes.

Sauteed Liver (flourless)

    3 tbsp. oil
    1 clove garlic
    1½ lbs. liver, cubed
    3 tbsp. nutritional yeast
    ¼ tsp. salt
    ½ tsp. marjoram

Heat the oil and saute the garlic. Remove the garlic and discard. Dredge the liver in the remaining ingredients. Saute 3 minutes on each side.

Boiled New England Dinner

    4 lbs. corned beef brisket
    4 peppercorns
    1 bay leaf
    ¼ tsp. thyme
    6 small potatoes, pared
    8 small white onions, peeled
    6 carrots, scraped
    1 small head of cabbage
    8 small turnips

Place meat in a large kettle with peppercorns, bay leaf and thyme and cover with cold water. Bring slowly to a boil and let simmer (covered) for 3-4 hours. Skim if necessary. With 45 minutes to go, add potatoes, onions and carrots and cook for 30 minutes. Cut cabbage into quarters and add it and the turnips to the top and cook 20 minutes longer. Place meat on a platter and vegetables around the side. Sprinkle parsley over the meat.

Lamb Sausage

5. lbs. lean, ground shoulder
1 tsp. cardamon seed
2 tsp. oregano
2 tsp. basil
½ cup leaf sage
2 tsp. papaya powder
1 tsp. thyme
1 tsp. marjoram

Mix together, shape into sausage patties and fry.

Fish Dishes

Baked Fish Omelet

4 egg yolks
½ cup milk
1 tsp. soy flour
2 cups, fish, cooked and flaked
1 tbsp. lemon juice
1 lemon rind
2 tbsp. oil
1 onion
½ green pepper
1 sprig parsley
2 tbsp. nutritional yeast
1 tsp. dulse
½ tsp. sage
4 egg whites beaten stiff

Put everything except egg whites into blender and blend until smooth. Pour into bowl. Fold-in stiffly beaten whites. Pour everything into an oiled pie plate and bake at 300 degrees until top is firm and dry—about 20 minutes.

Fish Casserole

½ cup fish (shrimp, crab, tuna)
1 cup finely diced celery
thin slices whole wheat bread
3 eggs, beaten
2½ cups milk
2 tsp. Worcestershire sauce
dash Tabasco

Alternate layers of fish and whole wheat bread in a 1½ qt.

casserole. Mix remainder of ingredients and pour over mixture. Bake in a 350 degree oven for 45 minutes.

Baked Fish Loaf

½ cup milk
1 egg, beaten
½ cup whole wheat flour
3 tbsp. soy flour
¼ cup soybeans, roasted, ground
2 cups fish, cooked, flaked
1 tsp. dulse, minced
3 tbsp. nutritional yeast
¼ tsp. ground nutmeg
½ cup grated cheddar cheese

Blend everything thoroughly. Turn into oiled loaf pan and bake at 350 degrees for an hour, until loaf is firm. Can be served hot or cold.

Salmon Patties

1 lb. canned, flaked salmon
¼ cup of dampened cornmeal
1 chopped onion
1 tsp. salt
½ tsp. pepper
½ cup tomato catsup
2 tbsp. lemon juice
1 egg, beaten
½ cup minced parsley

Drain liquid from salmon can into a measuring cup and add water to fill. Pour into saucepan, gradually adding cornmeal. Stir constantly. Cook over low heat until thick, then remove from flame. Mix salmon and rest of ingredients together in a bowl. Blend with the cornmeal mixture and form patties. Fry in hot oil until brown on both sides.

New England Bouillabaisse

½ cup salad oil
1 minced carrot
2 minced onions
1 clove garlic, minced
3 lbs. fish fillet
1 can tomato paste

1 can bouillon
2 cans clam chowder
1 doz. raw oysters
2 doz. shrimp, cooked and cleaned
¼ cup chopped parsley
2 tsp. salt
½ tsp. cayenned pepper
2 tbsp. lemon juice
½ cup canned shrimp soup

Heat the oil in a large skillet. Cook the carrots, onions and garlic for five minutes. Cut the fish fillets into small pieces and cook with the vegetables, also for 5 minutes. Add tomato paste, bouillon and clam chowder. Lower the heat and simmer for 15 minutes. Stir in shrimp, oysters, parsley and seasonings. Add shrimp soup. Heat and pour over buttered croutons.

Clam Casserole

2 cups milk
2 7 oz. cans minced clams
¼ cup minced onion
¼ tsp. pepper
24 whole wheat crackers
4 eggs, beaten
1 tsp. salt
¼ cup chopped parsley

Pour milk over the crackers. Add in the other ingredients and pour into a greased 1½ qt. casserole. Bake at 350 degrees for 45 minutes.

Vegetable Dishes

Eggplant Casserole

3 small eggplants
3 tbsp. oil
½ clove garlic minced
½ tsp. mint minced
1 cup cheese, grated
2 cups stewed tomatoes
1 onion, sliced
1 stalk celery and top, chopped

Wash eggplants with skins on. Slice into rounds ¼ inch thick. Saute in oil with garlic and mint. Arrange a layer of eggplant slices

in the bottom of an oiled casserole. Add a layer of cheese, tomatoes, onion and celery. Alternate layers until all ingredients are
used, topping with cheese. Bake at 350 degrees for about a half
hour.

Deep Dish Spinach Pie

2 lbs. spinach (raw, washed, and cut into bite size)
1 cup parsley sprigs, stems removed
1 cup green onions, chopped
¼ tsp. salt
½ tsp. rosemary
  nutmeg
2 tbsp. oil

Put ingredients in a pan and cook briefly, stirring once or twice
over low flame. Turn into oiled casserole. Cover with rolled
cheddar cheese piecrust. Bake 15 or 20 minutes at 425 degrees.

Zucchini Creole

4 zucchini
1 cup canned tomatoes
¼ cup chopped onions
1 small clove garlic, minced
2 tbsp. oil

Wash the zucchini and cut in lengthwise pieces. Place in saucepan with tomatoes, onions and garlic. Salt and pepper to taste.
Add oil and cover tightly. Bring to a boil, turn fire down to simmer
and cook 15 minutes. Serve with grated cheddar cheese.

Country Vegetable Stew

2 lb. cabbage
6 plump tomatoes
4 hard-boiled eggs
4 large spanish onions
2 cloves garlic
2 sticks celery
4 oz. melted butter
½ tsp. dill

Shred the cabbage finely, and cook in butter until tender. Add
the well-fried onions, celery and tomatoes. Mince the garlic and
mix into vegetables. Add the melted butter, dill and seasoning and

cook in a casserole in a slow oven for three quarters of an hour. Serve with sliced eggs on top.

Brussels Sprouts Casserole

1½ lbs. brussels sprouts, steamed
1 cup tomatoes stewed
½ cup cheddar cheese, grated
¼ tsp. nutmeg, grated
1 cup yogurt
½ cup roasted soybeans

Arrange sprouts in oiled casserole and cover with tomatoes. Sprinkle with cheese and nutmeg. Cover and bake at 350 degrees for 15 minutes. Serve garnished with yogurt and soy beans.

Baked Lima Beans

5 cups green lima beans
¼ lb. bacon cut small
1 cup tomato juice
¼ cup molasses
1 onion, grated
½ tsp. salt
3 tbsp. nutritional yeast
¼ tsp. sage

Mix all ingredients and turn into oiled casserole or bean pot. Cover and bake at 250 degrees for 2 to 3 hours. Leave uncovered during the last hour of baking.

Creamed Jerusalem Artichokes

1 lb. Jerusalem artichokes
4 oz. grated cheese
3 oz. butter
1 large, sweet spanish onion
whole wheat breadcrumbs

Steam the artichokes in a little salted water until tender. When cool enough to handle, rub off the skins and slice them into a shallow oven-proof dish. Cover with sliced onion, previously sauted in butter. Add a layer of cheese and a layer of breadcrumbs. Dot with butter, and brown in a hot oven for 10-15 minutes.

Sauteed Cabbage

4 cups shredded cabbage
3 tbsp. oil
1 tbsp. caraway seeds
2 cups sprouts

Saute cabbage briefly in oil, until it is slightly browned. Remove from the heat. Toss with seeds and sprouts.

Venezuelan Vegetable Pie

1 lb. hot mashed potatoes
1 lb. small diced potatoes
½ lb. freshly cooked peas
½ lb. shallots
1 egg yolk
2 tbsp. chopped chives
3 tbsp. butter
  mustard
  watercress

Steam the potatoes until tender. Ten minutes before they are done add peeled shallots. Then melt plenty of butter in a heavy skillet and saute the potatoes, shallots and peas until they are golden. Since the peas are precooked, this should take only a few minutes. Beat the chopped chives into the mashed potatoes and arrange them around the edge of your serving dish. Brush the potatoes with egg yolk, using all of it to make a heavy coating of egg. Heap the saute vegetables in the center and place under medium grill until potatoes begin to brown. Serve with the watercress.

These few recipes were only meant to give you an idea of how interesting, varied, and even *exciting*, healthy foods can be made. They need not be either bland or monotonous. For further natural recipes, consult the following books:

"Let's Cook It Right," Adelle Davis, 1970, Harcourt, Brace, Jovanovich.

"The Natural Foods Cookbook," Beatrice Trum Hunter, 1967, Simon & Schuster, Inc.

"International Vegetarian Cookery," Sonya Richmond, 1965, Arco Publishing.

"Hunza Health Secrets for Long Life and Happiness," Renee Taylor, 1964, Prentice-Hall, Inc.

"Eat, Drink, and Be Healthy," Agnes Toms, 1963, Devin-Adair Company.

SELECTED BIBLIOGRAPHY

Alsaker, Rasmus, M.D., "Victory Over Arthritis;" New York, Groton Press, 1966.

Bailey, Herbert, "Vitamin E; Your Key To a Healthy Heart;" New York, ARC Books, 1970.

Clark, Linda, A., M. A., "Secrets of Health and Beauty;" New York, Devin-Adair Company, 1969. "Stay Young Longer;" New York, Devin-Adair, 1968.

Davis, Adelle, "Let's Get Well;" New York, Harcourt, Brace & World, Inc., 1965. "Let's Cook It Right;" New York, Harcourt, Brace, Jovanovich, 1970.

Elwood, Catharyn, "Feel Like A Million;" New York, Devin-Adair, 1965.

Hunter, Beatrice Trum, "The Natural Foods Cookbook;" New York, Simon & Schuster, Inc., 1967.

Jarvis, D. C., M.D., "Folk Medicine;" Greenwich, Conn., Fawcett Publications, 1961.

Knutson, Gunilla, "Beauty and Health the Scandinavian Way;" New York, Avon Books, 1969.

La Lanne, Jack, "Foods For Glamour;" New York, Arc Books Inc., 1961.

MacFadyen, Ralph J., "See Without Glasses;" Greenwich, Conn., Fawcett Publications, 1966.

Rawls, Eugene and Diskin, Eve, "Yoga For Beauty and Health;" New York, Prentice-Hall, Inc., 1967.

Richardson, R. A., M.D., "Facial Wrinkles;" Mokelumna Hill, Calif., Health Research, 1964.

Richmond, Sonya, "International Vegetarian Cookery;" New York, Arco Publishing, 1965.

Rutledge, Deborah, "Natural Beauty Secrets;" New York, Avon Books, 1966.

Schultz, Dodi, "The ABC's of Skin Care;" New York, Bantam Books, 1969. "Have Your Baby and Your Figure Too;" New York, Hawthorne Books, 1970.

Shelton, Herbert M., "Food Combining Made Easy;" San Antonio, Texas, Dr. Shelton's Health School, 1964.

Taylor, Renee, "Hunza Health Secrets;" New Jersey, Prentice-Hall, Inc., 1964.

Toms, Agnes, "Eat, Drink, and Be Healthy;" New York, Devin-Adair Company, 1968.

Vannier, Maryhelen, "A Better Figure For You;" New York, Tower Publications, 1965.

Vishnudevananda, Swami, "The Complete Illustrated Book of Yoga;" New York, Julian Press, 1960.

Wade, Carlson, "The Natural Way to Health and Beauty;" New York, Bantam Books, 1968.

Warmbrand, Max, M.D., "The Encyclopedia of Natural Health;" Island Park, New York, Groton Press, 1967.

INDEX